UNDERSTANDING

DEMENTIA

General Knowledge on Dementia; A Manual
for Relatives, Companions, and Care
Providers

DISCLAIMER

The book *"Understanding Dementia"* serves as a supplementary resource rather than a substitute for medical consultation and diagnostic evaluation. Its primary purpose is to impart general knowledge about the disease and offer guidance on the care and management of patients, emphasising the importance of obtaining a formal diagnosis from a healthcare professional.

Table of Contents

Chapter 1: Understanding Dementia

What Is Dementia?

Dementia is not a specific disease but rather a broad term used to describe a group of cognitive impairments that affect memory, thinking, and daily functioning. It is characterised by a decline in cognitive abilities that goes beyond what is considered a normal part of ageing and interferes with a person's ability to carry out daily activities.

Common symptoms of Dementia may include:

1. **Memory Loss:** Individuals with dementia often have difficulty remembering recent events, names, and conversations.

2. **Difficulty with Communication:** This can involve difficulty finding the right words, following or joining in conversations, and understanding what others are saying.

3. **Impaired Reasoning and Judgement:** People with dementia may have trouble making decisions,

solving problems, or handling complex tasks.

4. **Changes in Visual Perception:** This can include difficulty recognising familiar faces or objects, as well as problems with spatial orientation.

5. **Personality and Behaviour Changes:** Dementia can lead to mood swings, personality changes, agitation, and even aggression in some cases.

6. **Disorientation:** Individuals with dementia may become confused about time, place, and identity.

7. **Impaired Motor Skills:** As dementia progresses, coordination and motor skills may decline, making it difficult to perform tasks such as dressing and grooming.

There are several different types of dementia, with Alzheimer's disease being the most common. Other types include vascular dementia, Lewy body dementia, frontotemporal dementia, and more. Each type has distinct characteristics and underlying causes.

The exact cause of dementia varies depending on the type, but it often involves damage or degeneration of brain cells and neural pathways. Age is a significant risk factor for dementia, and the condition becomes more prevalent as people get older. However, it's important to note that dementia is not a normal part of ageing, and not all older adults develop it.

Early diagnosis and appropriate management can help individuals with dementia and their families better cope with the condition and improve their quality of life. Treatment approaches may include medications, cognitive rehabilitation, behavioural interventions, and support services. The progression and prognosis of dementia vary widely depending on the underlying cause and individual factors.

Types of Dementia

Dementia is a broad term used to describe a range of cognitive impairments that interfere with a person's daily functioning. There are several different types of dementia, each with its distinct characteristics and causes. Some of the most common types of dementia include the following:

1. **Alzheimer's Disease:** Alzheimer's disease is the most common type of dementia, accounting for the majority of cases. It is characterised by the progressive deterioration of memory, thinking, and behaviour. Plaques and tangles in the brain are hallmarks of this disease. Alzheimer's disease is a degenerative neurological condition that impairs thinking abilities, behaviour, and memory. Dementia, a term used to describe memory loss and other cognitive impairments severe enough to impede day-to-day

functioning, is most commonly caused by it. Alzheimer's disease progressively deteriorates over time, impairing cognitive function and ultimately making it impossible to do even the most basic tasks. The exact cause of Alzheimer's disease is not yet fully understood, but it is believed to involve a combination of genetic, environmental, and lifestyle factors. Some of the hallmarks of Alzheimer's include the buildup of certain proteins in the brain, such as beta-amyloid plaques and tau tangles, which interfere with communication between nerve cells and eventually lead to cell death. Symptoms of Alzheimer's disease typically develop slowly and worsen over time. They can vary from person to person but often include memory loss, confusion, difficulty with problem-solving or language, changes in mood or behaviour, and eventually a loss of ability to recognise loved ones or perform basic tasks. Although there isn't a cure for Alzheimer's disease at this time, there are therapies that can help some people manage their symptoms and live better lives. Future understanding and treatment of this debilitating ailment could be improved with more research into possible remedies and preventive strategies.

2. **Vascular Dementia:** Vascular dementia is another common type of dementia, and it's caused by damage to the brain's blood vessels. This damage impairs blood flow to brain tissue, leading to problems with thinking, reasoning, and memory. The

risk factors for vascular dementia are similar to those for heart disease and stroke, including high blood pressure, high cholesterol, diabetes, smoking, and obesity. These factors can damage blood vessels in the brain, leading to strokes or mini-strokes (transient ischemic attacks) that can result in vascular dementia. Depending on the degree and location of brain damage, vascular dementia symptoms can vary greatly, but they frequently involve behavioural and emotional changes along with problems with memory, thinking, and judgement. Since vascular dementia frequently develops gradually after each stroke or vascular incident, its course can be more unpredictable than that of Alzheimer's disease. The diagnosis of vascular dementia typically involves a thorough medical history, physical examination, cognitive testing, and sometimes brain imaging studies such as MRI or CT scans. Treatment focuses on managing underlying risk factors, such as controlling blood pressure and cholesterol levels, as well as addressing symptoms to improve quality of life. Preventing vascular dementia involves maintaining a healthy lifestyle, including regular exercise, a balanced diet, not smoking, and managing conditions like high blood pressure and diabetes. Early detection and management of risk factors can help reduce the risk of developing vascular dementia later in life.

3. **Lewy Body Dementia:** Lewy body dementia (LBD) is a progressive brain disorder that affects thinking,

behaviour, and movement. It's characterised by the presence of abnormal protein deposits called Lewy bodies in the brain. These deposits disrupt the normal functioning of brain cells, leading to a decline in cognitive abilities and motor control. Lewy body dementia shares some similarities with both Alzheimer's disease and Parkinson's disease. Like Alzheimer's, it can cause memory loss, confusion, and other cognitive symptoms. Like Parkinson's, it can cause movement problems such as tremors, stiffness, and impaired balance. Individual differences in LBD symptoms are common, as is their tendency to change in intensity. REM sleep behaviour disorder (acting out dreams while asleep), visual hallucinations, changes in alertness and concentration, and autonomic dysfunction (disorders involving blood pressure, heart rate, and digestion) are among the other symptoms that people with LBD may encounter in addition to cognitive and motor symptoms. Diagnosing LBD can be challenging because its symptoms overlap with those of other conditions, particularly Alzheimer's disease and Parkinson's disease. A comprehensive evaluation by a neurologist or other specialist familiar with LBD is usually necessary to make an accurate diagnosis. There is currently no cure for LBD, but treatment focuses on managing symptoms to improve quality of life. This may include medications to address cognitive symptoms, movement problems, and psychiatric symptoms like depression or hallucinations. Supportive therapies such as physical therapy, occupational therapy, and speech therapy can also be helpful.

LBD can have a substantial impact on patients and the people who care for them, thus information, education, and emotional support are offered to those who are impacted by the illness through support groups and other services. Lewy body dementia patients and their families may find it easier to deal with the difficulties of having the disease if it is diagnosed and treated early.

4. **Frontotemporal Dementia (FTD):** Frontotemporal dementia (FTD) is a group of disorders caused by progressive nerve cell loss in the brain's frontal lobes (the areas behind the forehead) and/or its temporal lobes (the areas behind the ears). This loss of nerve cells leads to changes in personality, behaviour, and language skills. FTD typically affects individuals in their 40s, 50s, and 60s, although it can occur at later ages as well. The

exact cause of FTD is not fully understood, but it is believed to involve a combination of genetic, environmental, and other factors.

There are several subtypes of FTD, each with its own characteristic symptoms:

- Behavioural variant frontotemporal dementia (bvFTD): This subtype is characterised by changes in behaviour, personality, and social conduct. Individuals may exhibit disinhibition, apathy, loss of empathy, compulsive behaviours, and poor judgement.

- Primary progressive aphasia (PPA):
  This subtype primarily affects
  language abilities. Individuals may
  have difficulty speaking,
  understanding language, or finding
  words. There are three variants of
  PPA: the nonfluent/agrammatic
  variant, the semantic variant, and the
  logopenic variant.
- Semantic dementia: This subtype is
  characterised by the loss of the
  meaning of words and objects.
  Individuals may have difficulty
  understanding and naming objects

and may exhibit changes in social behaviour.

- Progressive supranuclear palsy (PSP) and corticobasal syndrome (CBS): These are two related movement disorders that are sometimes considered part of the FTD spectrum. PSP typically involves problems with balance, eye movement, and walking, while CBS involves symptoms such as stiffness, tremors, and difficulty with voluntary movements.

Since the symptoms of FTD can mimic those of other illnesses like psychiatric disorders and Alzheimer's disease, diagnosing the disease can be difficult. To achieve an accurate diagnosis, a thorough evaluation, including neurological examination, cognitive tests, and brain imaging, by a neurologist or other professional experienced with FTD is typically required. Since there is presently no known cure for FTD, the main goals of treatment are to manage symptoms and offer individuals and their families support. This could involve taking medicine for behavioural symptoms, getting speech therapy for language issues, and receiving supportive care for both emotional and physical needs. Future improvements in diagnosis and therapy are possible because of continuing research into possible therapies and biomarkers for FTD.

5. **Mixed Dementia:** Some individuals may have a combination of two or more types of dementia. For example, someone may have both Alzheimer's disease and vascular dementia simultaneously, leading to mixed dementia.

6. **Creutzfeldt-Jakob Disease (CJD):** Creutzfeldt-Jakob disease (CJD) is a rare, degenerative brain

disorder that leads to rapid neurological decline. It belongs to a group of diseases known as prion diseases, which occur when abnormal proteins called prions accumulate in the brain, causing damage to nerve cells.

CJD can occur in several forms, including:

- **Sporadic CJD:** This is the most common form, accounting for about 85% of cases. It occurs spontaneously and without any known cause.

- **Familial or inherited CJD:** In some cases, CJD can be inherited due

to mutations in the PRNP gene, which
provides instructions for making the
prion protein. This form accounts for
about 10-15% of cases.

- **Acquired CJD:** This form occurs as a
  result of exposure to contaminated
  tissues, such as through medical
  procedures (iatrogenic CJD) or
  consumption of contaminated food
  products (variant CJD). Variant CJD
  is linked to the consumption of beef
  products contaminated with the prion
  responsible for bovine spongiform

encephalopathy (BSE), also known as "mad cow disease."

Rapidly progressing dementia and alterations in behaviour, cognition, coordination, and vision are common symptoms of CJD. People may have muscle rigidity, uncontrollable movements, and trouble speaking and walking as the illness worsens. Most patients pass away from the condition within months to a few years following the commencement of symptoms, indicating how quickly the illness progresses. Because the symptoms of CJD can mimic those of other neurological conditions, diagnosing the condition can be difficult. Finding aberrant prions frequently entails clinical assessment, electroencephalography (EEG), brain imaging (MRI), and sometimes a brain sample or cerebrospinal fluid investigation. Since there isn't a cure for CJD yet, supportive care and symptom relief are the main goals of treatment. The disease is usually deadly, so the prognosis is not good. To prevent acquired forms of CJD, precautions must be taken to avoid contact with contaminated tissues. These precautions include making sure medical procedures are safe, and putting laws in place to stop prion diseases from spreading to the food supply.

7. **Huntington's Disease:** Huntington's disease (HD) is a hereditary neurological disorder that leads to progressive degeneration of nerve cells in the brain. It is caused by a mutation in the HTT gene, which provides instructions for making a protein called huntingtin. The mutated form of the protein leads to damage in specific areas of the brain, particularly the basal ganglia and

cerebral cortex. HD is inherited in an autosomal dominant pattern, meaning that a person only needs to inherit one copy of the mutated gene from either parent to develop the disease. If a parent has the HD gene mutation, each child has a 50% chance of inheriting it. HD symptoms can manifest at any age, however, they typically start between the ages of 30 and 50. The defining characteristic of Huntington's disease (HD) is the uncontrollable movements, or chorea, that might include jerking or writhing of the body, face, and limbs. Additional symptoms include issues with speech, swallowing, and coordination, as well as changes in mood, personality, and cognitive function. People with HD may experience deteriorating physical and cognitive symptoms as the disease advances, which can result in considerable impairment and the ultimate need for full-time care. The pace at which a disease progresses can differ significantly between people. A combination of clinical assessment, genetic testing to identify the HTT gene mutation, and symptom assessment is usually used to diagnose HD. HD currently has no known cure; supportive care and symptom management are the mainstays of treatment. While therapy and support groups can offer people and their families practical help and emotional support, medications can help reduce some of the physical and psychological symptoms related to the illness. There is currently a great deal of research being done on possible treatments for

HD, including developing disease-modifying medications that would stop or delay the disease's progression. For those who are at risk of HD or have a family history of the condition, genetic testing and counselling are offered to help them make decisions about their health and future.

8. **Wernicke-Korsakoff Syndrome:** Wernicke-Korsakoff syndrome (WKS) is a neurological disorder caused by a severe deficiency of thiamine (vitamin B1), which is essential for proper brain

function. It is most commonly associated with chronic alcohol abuse, although it can also occur in other conditions that lead to thiamine deficiency, such as malnutrition, gastrointestinal surgery, or prolonged vomiting.

Wernicke's encephalopathy is the acute phase of the disorder and is characterised by a triad of symptoms:

- Confusion and changes in mental status
- Ataxia (loss of coordination)

- Ophthalmoplegia (paralysis or weakness of the muscles that control eye movement)

Wernicke's encephalopathy can lead to Korsakoff syndrome if treatment is not received; this condition is characterised by significant memory loss, confabulation (making up stories to fill in memory gaps), and other cognitive impairments. Apart from these symptoms, people with Korsakoff syndrome might also display apathy, personality changes, and problems with insight and judgement. Blood tests to measure thiamine levels are frequently used in conjunction with clinical evaluation, which includes a comprehensive medical history and physical examination, to diagnose Wernicke-Korsakoff syndrome. MRIs and other forms of brain imaging tests may also be carried out to check for indications of brain injury. Treatment for Wernicke-Korsakoff syndrome involves the administration of thiamine supplements, usually given intravenously to ensure rapid absorption. In addition to thiamine supplementation, individuals may require nutritional support and rehabilitation to address any physical or cognitive deficits.

Wernicke-Korsakoff syndrome must be identified and treated as soon as possible to enhance results and avoid irreversible brain damage. Nonetheless, some people may continue to have cognitive and functional impairments despite receiving treatment. To prevent Wernicke-Korsakoff syndrome, risk factors like alcohol misuse and inadequate nutrition must be addressed, especially in populations where thiamine deficiency is more common.

9. **Parkinson's Disease Dementia:** The term "Parkinson's disease dementia" (PDD) describes the

progressive cognitive deterioration and dementia that can occur in people with Parkinson's disease (PD). Parkinson's disease is a degenerative neurological condition marked by tremors, stiffness, slowness of movement, and imbalance problems. Although movement is the primary symptom of Parkinson's disease, cognitive symptoms can also arise, particularly in the latter stages of the disease. These symptoms include disorientation, memory loss, and problems with executive function, which includes organising, planning, and problem-solving. It is commonly referred to as Parkinson's disease dementia when these cognitive symptoms worsen to the point where they substantially impair day-to-day functioning. The exact cause of PDD is not fully understood, but it is believed to involve a combination of factors, including the accumulation of abnormal proteins in the brain, such as alpha-synuclein, which is also implicated in the motor symptoms of Parkinson's disease. Other factors, such as changes in neurotransmitter levels and inflammation in the brain, may also contribute to cognitive decline in PD.

A comprehensive medical evaluation, which includes a review of symptoms, cognitive testing, and occasionally brain imaging investigations like MRIs or CT scans, is necessary to diagnose PDD. It's critical to differentiate PDD from other dementia causes, such as vascular dementia or Alzheimer's disease, which might coexist with PD or have symptoms that match. PDD treatment emphasises symptom management and quality of life enhancement. This could involve therapies including physical therapy, occupational therapy, and speech therapy to address motor and cognitive impairments, as well as drugs to regulate behavioural symptoms and enhance cognitive performance. Other crucial elements of managing PDD include education, carer support, and supportive interventions. While there is currently no cure for PDD, ongoing research aims to better understand the underlying mechanisms of cognitive decline in PD and develop more effective treatments. Strategies to promote brain health, such as regular exercise, a healthy diet, and cognitive stimulation, may also help to support cognitive function in individuals with Parkinson's disease.

10. **Normal Pressure Hydrocephalus (NPH):** Normal pressure hydrocephalus (NPH) is a neurological condition characterised by the abnormal accumulation of

cerebrospinal fluid (CSF) in the brain's ventricles, leading to the enlargement of these fluid-filled cavities. Despite the increased fluid volume, the pressure inside the skull remains within the normal range, hence the name "normal pressure" hydrocephalus.

The exact cause of NPH is often unknown, but it can result from various factors such as infections, haemorrhage, head injury, brain tumour, or certain neurological conditions. In some cases, NPH may develop spontaneously without an identifiable cause.

NPH typically affects older adults, with symptoms usually appearing in individuals over the age of 60. The classic triad of symptoms associated with NPH includes:

- **Gait disturbances:** Individuals may experience difficulty walking, characterised by a wide-based, shuffling gait with short, hesitant steps. They may also exhibit balance problems and a tendency to fall backward.

- **Cognitive impairment:** Mild cognitive impairment is common in NPH, with individuals experiencing problems with memory, attention, and executive function (planning, organising, and problem-solving).

- **Urinary incontinence:** Many individuals with NPH develop urinary urgency, frequency, or incontinence, which may be one of the earliest symptoms.

Since the symptoms of NPH might mimic those of other neurological disorders like Parkinson's disease or Alzheimer's disease, diagnosing NPH can be difficult. Clinical assessment, neuroimaging examinations (MRIs, CT scans), and CSF pressure and flow measurements are frequently combined in this process. Surgery is usually required as part of NPH treatment to remove extra CSF from the brain and reduce pressure on brain tissue. Installing a ventriculoperitoneal shunt, which directs CSF from the brain's ventricles to the abdominal cavity, where it can be absorbed by the body, is the most often performed surgical surgery for NPH. While many NPH patients find that having a shunt placed improves their quality of life and symptoms, not everyone responds to surgery, and some people may continue to have symptoms even after receiving therapy. To control potential issues related to shunt installation and optimise outcomes, close monitoring and follow-up are crucial.

11. **Posterior Cortical Atrophy (PCA):** Posterior cortical atrophy (PCA) is a rare neurodegenerative condition characterised by progressive degeneration of the brain's posterior cortex, which includes the regions responsible for visual processing, spatial awareness, and attention. PCA is often considered a variant of Alzheimer's disease, although it can

also be associated with other underlying causes, such as Lewy body dementia or Creutzfeldt-Jakob disease. PCA usually strikes people in their 50s or 60s, while it can start earlier or later in life. Visual disturbances, including problems with reading, identifying persons or objects, estimating distances, and navigating through space, are the most prevalent first symptoms of PCA. As the illness worsens, more cognitive symptoms like memory loss, language problems, and executive dysfunction (organising, planning, and problem-solving) may appear.

It can be difficult to diagnose PCA since its symptoms might be confused with those of other neurodegenerative diseases, especially early-onset Alzheimer's disease or dementias containing Lewy bodies. To determine the structure and function of the brain, a comprehensive medical assessment is frequently conducted, which includes a review of symptoms, cognitive tests, and neuroimaging procedures (such as MRI or PET scans). There is currently no cure for PCA, and treatment focuses on managing symptoms and optimising quality of life. This may include strategies to address visual difficulties, such as using assistive devices, modifying the environment, and providing rehabilitation services. Medications to manage cognitive symptoms or behavioural changes may also be prescribed, although their effectiveness can vary among individuals. Supportive care and education for individuals with PCA and their carers are essential components of management. This may involve accessing resources such as support groups, counselling services, and community organisations that specialise in dementia care. Ongoing research into the underlying causes and mechanisms of PCA may lead to improved diagnostic tools and therapeutic interventions in the future.

Remember that the underlying cause of dementia can have a significant impact on the specific symptoms and course of the disease. For those who have dementia and their families, an accurate diagnosis, and suitable care are essential. Seeking medical attention and assistance from healthcare specialists is crucial if you or a loved one is exhibiting signs of dementia.

Common Symptoms

Dementia is a broad term that refers to a variety of mental disorders that interfere with a person's everyday functioning and quality of life. The following are common dementia symptoms:

1. **Memory Loss:** Difficulty remembering recent events, names, and important details.

2. **Disorientation:** Confusion about time, place, and people.

3. **Impaired Communication:** Difficulty finding the right words, expressing thoughts, or following conversations.

4. **Poor Judgement and Decision-making:** Making uncharacteristic choices or struggling to make sound decisions.

5. **Difficulty with Complex Tasks:** Struggling with tasks that involve multiple steps, such as cooking or managing finances.

6. **Problems with Abstract Thinking:** Difficulty with concepts like time or money.

7. **Misplacing Things:** Frequently losing belongings and being unable to retrace steps to find them.

8. **Changes in Mood or Behaviour:** Exhibiting mood swings, irritability, and personality changes.

9. **Decreased Visual and Spatial Abilities:** Difficulty with tasks that require visual perception and spatial awareness, like driving.

10. **Decreased Motor Skills:** Struggles with coordination, balance, and physical activities.

11. **Social Withdrawal:** Isolation and withdrawal from social activities and relationships.

12. **Reduced Self-care:** Neglecting personal hygiene, nutrition, and other self-care tasks.

13.**Repetitive Behaviours**: Engaging in repetitive actions, such as pacing or asking the same questions.

14.**Agitation and Restlessness:** Feeling anxious, restless, or easily upset.

15.**Hallucinations or Delusions:** Experiencing false sensory perceptions or beliefs.

16.**Sleep Disturbances:** Disrupted sleep patterns, including insomnia or daytime drowsiness.

It's important to note that dementia is not a normal part of ageing. While these symptoms can be associated with various types of dementia, such as Alzheimer's disease, Lewy body dementia, vascular dementia, and frontotemporal dementia, they can also be caused by other medical conditions. If you or someone you know is experiencing these symptoms, it's essential to consult a healthcare professional for a proper evaluation and diagnosis. Early diagnosis and appropriate care can help manage the condition and improve the quality of life for individuals with dementia and their caregivers.

Causes and Risk Factors

Dementia is a complex condition with various potential causes and risk factors. The specific cause of dementia can vary depending on the type of dementia. Some common causes and risk factors for dementia include:

1. **Age:** Advancing age is the most significant risk factor for most types of dementia. The risk of dementia increases as people get older, especially after the age of 65.

2. **Alzheimer's Disease:** Alzheimer's disease is the most common cause of

dementia, and is characterised by the accumulation of amyloid plaques and tau tangles in the brain.

3. **Genetics:** A family history of dementia can increase the risk of developing the condition. Some types of dementia have a strong genetic component.

4. **Down Syndrome:** People with Down syndrome are at a higher risk of developing Alzheimer's disease and other forms of dementia.

5. **Vascular Factors:** Conditions that affect the blood vessels, such as

hypertension, diabetes, and high cholesterol, can contribute to vascular dementia, which is caused by impaired blood flow to the brain.

6. **Brain Injuries:** Traumatic brain injuries, such as those from a concussion or repeated head trauma (as seen in some athletes), can lead to long-term cognitive impairment.

7. **Stroke:** A history of strokes or mini-strokes (transient ischemic attacks) can increase the risk of vascular dementia.

8. **Other Medical Conditions:** Some medical conditions, like Parkinson's disease, Huntington's disease, and Creutzfeldt-Jakob disease, can lead to specific types of dementia.

9. **Lifestyle Factors:** Unhealthy lifestyle choices, such as a lack of physical activity, poor diet, smoking, and excessive alcohol consumption, may increase the risk of dementia.

10. **Environmental Factors:** Long-term exposure to certain environmental toxins or pollution may

contribute to the development of dementia.

11. **Social and Educational Factors:** Lower levels of education and limited social engagement have been associated with a higher risk of dementia.

12. **Depression and Mental Health:** Chronic depression, anxiety, and other mental health conditions can be risk factors for cognitive decline and dementia.

13. **Poor Cardiovascular Health:** Cardiovascular risk factors, such as

high blood pressure, obesity, and heart disease, can also increase the risk of dementia.

14. **Hormonal Changes:** Some research suggests that hormonal changes, such as those that occur during menopause, may be associated with an increased risk of certain types of dementia.

It's vital to remember that not every dementia case has a single, obvious cause or risk factor. A multitude of variables can lead to dementia, and the underlying mechanisms are still poorly understood. Dementia risk can be decreased by reducing risk factors with a healthy lifestyle, controlling chronic diseases, and engaging in mental and physical activities. For dementia to be effectively managed and treated, early detection and intervention are essential.

Chapter 2: The Journey Begins

Early Signs and Diagnosis

Effective management and treatment of dementia depend on early diagnosis and identification. Early dementia symptoms and indicators can help people and their families seek medical attention and support. Typical early dementia symptoms include the following:

1. **Memory Loss:** Forgetfulness, particularly related to recent events, appointments, or conversations, is a common early sign of dementia.

2. **Difficulty with Familiar Tasks:**
   Individuals may struggle with tasks
   they used to perform easily, such as
   cooking, dressing, or using household
   appliances.

3. **Language Problems:** Difficulty
   finding the right words, repeating
   oneself, or struggling to follow or
   participate in conversations can be
   early signs.

4. **Disorientation:** Getting lost in
   familiar places, losing track of time, or
   not recognising familiar faces or
   locations.

5. **Poor Judgement:** Making poor decisions, demonstrating impaired judgement, or engaging in risky behaviour.

6. **Problems with Planning and Organizing:** Difficulty with tasks that involve multiple steps, such as managing finances, planning events, or organising activities.

7. **Misplacing Items:** Frequently misplacing belongings and being unable to retrace steps to find them

8. **Mood and Personality Changes:** Experiencing mood swings,

irritability, or personality changes that are unusual for the person

9. **Social Withdrawal:** Becoming increasingly isolated and withdrawing from social activities or relationships

10. **Decreased Interest in Hobbies:** Losing interest in hobbies or activities that were once enjoyable.

11. **Changes in Visual and Spatial Abilities:** Difficulty with tasks that require visual perception and spatial awareness, like driving.

12. **Repetitive Behaviours:** Engaging

in repetitive actions, such as pacing or

asking the same questions.

It is noteworthy that certain symptoms may

also arise from non-dementia-related

diseases, including depression,

pharmaceutical side effects, or other

medical problems. A thorough assessment

by a medical specialist is required to get an

accurate diagnosis and identify the reason

behind these symptoms. Typically, the

dementia diagnosis procedure entails:

1. **Medical History:** The doctor will

ask about the individual's medical

history, including any family history of dementia.

2. **Physical Examination:** A physical examination helps rule out other medical conditions that may be causing the symptoms.

3. **Cognitive Assessment:** Cognitive tests and assessments, such as the Mini-Mental State Examination (MMSE) or the Montreal Cognitive Assessment (MoCA), can help assess cognitive function.

4. **Brain Imaging:** Brain imaging studies, such as MRI or CT scans, may

be used to identify structural changes in the brain.

5. **Blood Tests:** Blood tests can help rule out other medical conditions, such as vitamin deficiencies, thyroid dysfunction, or infections.

6. **Neuropsychological Testing:** More detailed neuropsychological assessments may be conducted to evaluate specific cognitive functions.

7. **Functional Assessment:** Evaluating a person's ability to perform daily tasks and activities of daily living

8. **Consultation with Specialists:**
   Depending on the results, further consultation with specialists, such as neurologists or geriatricians may be necessary.

Early diagnosis allows for the implementation of interventions, treatment, and support services to manage the condition and improve the individual's quality of life. It also enables individuals and their families to plan for the future and make informed decisions about care and support.

Navigating the Diagnostic Process

Although navigating the dementia diagnostic process can be difficult, doing so is essential to comprehending the illness and receiving the right support and care. Here is a roadmap to help you through this procedure:

Recognise Early Signs: As mentioned earlier, recognising early signs and symptoms of dementia is the first step. If you or a loved one is experiencing these signs, it's essential to seek medical evaluation.

Consult with a Healthcare Professional: Start by scheduling an appointment with a primary care physician or a geriatrician. They can conduct an initial assessment and may refer you to specialists if needed.

Prepare for the Appointment:

- Create a list of the specific symptoms and changes you've noticed, including when they started.

- Provide information about your medical history and any family history of dementia.

- Bring a list of current
  medications and supplements.

- Be prepared to discuss any
  recent illnesses or significant life
  events.

Medical Evaluation:

- The healthcare professional will
  perform a physical examination
  to rule out other medical
  conditions.

- Cognitive assessments and tests,
  such as the Mini-Mental State
  Examination (MMSE) or the

Montreal Cognitive Assessment (MoCA), may be administered.

- Blood tests can help identify reversible causes of cognitive impairment, like vitamin deficiencies or thyroid issues.

Brain Imaging:

- Depending on the findings, the doctor may recommend brain imaging studies, such as MRI or CT scans, to look for structural changes in the brain.

Neuropsychological Assessment:

- More detailed neuropsychological testing may be conducted to assess specific cognitive functions.

Consultation with Specialists:

- If the initial evaluations suggest a possible diagnosis of dementia, you may be referred to specialists like neurologists, geriatric psychiatrists, or neuropsychologists for further assessment.

Support for Caregivers:

- Carers and family members should also seek support and education on dementia. Local support groups, organisations like the Alzheimer's Association, or mental health professionals can offer valuable guidance and resources.

Receive a Diagnosis:

- Once the diagnostic process is complete, the healthcare professional will provide a

diagnosis, which may include
the type and stage of dementia.

Care and Planning:

- After a diagnosis, it's important
  to discuss a care plan and
  treatment options with the
  healthcare team. This may
  include medications, lifestyle
  modifications, and access to
  support services.

Legal and Financial Planning:

- Consult an attorney or financial
  planner to address legal and
  financial matters, such as estate

planning, power of attorney, and long-term care options.

Emotional Support:

- A dementia diagnosis can be emotionally challenging for both the individual and their family. Seek emotional support from friends, family, or mental health professionals.

Explore Available Resources:

- Learn about local and national resources that can provide information, support, and respite care. These may include day programs, in-home care services, and caregiver support groups.

Create a Care Team:

- Develop a team of healthcare professionals, including the primary care physician, specialists, and caregivers, to coordinate care and address the evolving needs of the person with dementia.

Monitor and Adjust:

- Dementia is a progressive condition, so regular check-ups

and ongoing monitoring are important. The care plan may need to be adjusted as the condition changes.

Remember that a dementia diagnosis is not the end but the beginning of a journey. With appropriate care, support, and planning, individuals with dementia and their families can maximise their quality of life and manage the challenges associated with the condition.

Emotional Impact on Patients and Families

Dementia has a profound emotional impact on both patients and their families. Coping with the diagnosis and the progression of the disease can be emotionally challenging and may lead to a range of emotions and experiences. Here are some of the emotional impacts on patients and families:

Emotional Impact on Patients:

1. **Confusion and Frustration:** Dementia often causes individuals to become confused, frustrated, and

anxious as they struggle with memory loss and difficulties in daily life.

2. **Depression:** Many people with dementia experience depression due to their awareness of cognitive decline and the challenges they face.

3. **Loss of Identity:** Dementia can erode a person's sense of self as they struggle to recognise themselves and their history.

4. **Isolation:** Communication difficulties and cognitive decline can lead to social isolation, making individuals with dementia feel

disconnected from friends and loved ones.

5. **Agitation and Aggression:** Some individuals may exhibit behaviours like agitation, aggression, or restlessness due to their frustration and inability to express their needs.

Emotional Impact on Families:

1. **Grief and Loss:** Family members often experience grief and a sense of loss as they witness their loved one's decline. They grieve for the person they used to know.

2. **Stress and Caregiver Burnout:**
   Caring for someone with dementia can be physically and emotionally exhausting. Caregivers may experience high levels of stress and burnout.

3. **Financial Stress:** The cost of dementia care, including medical expenses and caregiving services, can create significant financial stress for families.

4. **Feelings of Helplessness:** Families may feel powerless in the face of a progressive disease for which there is currently no cure.

5. **Relationship Strain:** Dementia can strain relationships within families as roles and responsibilities shift, and communication becomes more challenging.

6. **Stigma and Isolation:** Some families may experience social stigma and isolation due to misconceptions and misunderstandings about dementia.

7. **Mixed Emotions:** Family members often experience a mix of love, compassion, frustration, guilt, and sadness as they navigate the

complexities of caring for someone with dementia.

8. **Long-Term Stress:** Dementia can be a long-term, chronic condition, which means that families may experience stress and emotional burdens for an extended period.

Both patients and families need to seek emotional support and resources to help manage these emotional challenges. Support groups, counselling, and education about dementia can be invaluable in helping individuals and families cope with the emotional impact of the disease. Creating a supportive care network and ensuring self-care for caregivers is essential to maintaining the well-being of both the individuals with dementia and their loved ones. Additionally, understanding and compassion from the community and healthcare professionals can make a significant difference in addressing the emotional impact of dementia on patients and families.

Chapter 3: Care and Support

Building a Supportive Network

Caring for individuals living with dementia requires a comprehensive approach that involves building a supportive network of professionals, family members, and friends. Here are some key steps to provide care and support for patients with dementia and create a strong support network:

Educate Yourself: Understand the specific type of dementia the person has been diagnosed with and the stage of the disease. Learn about its symptoms, progression, and how it affects cognitive and physical function.

Consult Healthcare Professionals:

- Work closely with healthcare professionals, including the primary care physician, neurologist, geriatrician, and dementia specialists.

- Seek guidance on treatment options, medications, and non-pharmacological interventions.

Involve the Person with Dementia:

- Encourage their involvement in decisions about their care and preferences.
- Respect their dignity, autonomy, and independence to the extent possible.

Build a Care Team:

- Establish a multidisciplinary care team, including doctors, nurses, social workers, and therapists, to provide comprehensive care.

- Consider specialised dementia care programs or memory clinics.

Create a Safe Environment:

- Modify the living space to reduce hazards and enhance safety.
- Install locks, alarms, and other safety measures to prevent wandering.

Develop a Routine:

- Establish a daily routine to provide structure and predictability.

- Consistency in daily activities can reduce anxiety and confusion.

Communication:

- Use clear and simple language when communicating with a person with dementia.

- Be patient and offer reassurance during moments of confusion or frustration.

Behavioural Management:

- Learn how to manage challenging behaviours, such as agitation or aggression, with techniques like redirection, validation therapy, and music therapy.

Take Part in Mental Tasks:

- Provide mentally stimulating activities, like puzzles, games, and reminiscence therapy, to maintain cognitive function and promote social interaction.

Nutrition and Hydration:

- Ensure the person with dementia is receiving a balanced diet and staying adequately hydrated.

- Address any dietary restrictions or difficulties with swallowing.

Medication Management:

- Work closely with healthcare professionals to manage medications, and be aware of potential side effects and interactions.

Respite Care:

- Arrange for respite care to give family caregivers a break from caregiving responsibilities.

Legal and Financial Planning

- Address legal and financial
  matters, including powers of
  attorney, advance directives, and
  long-term care planning.

Support Groups:

- Join support groups for
  caregivers and people with
  dementia to share experiences
  and receive emotional support
  and practical advice.

Home Care Services:

- Consider in-home care services,
  such as home health aides or

nursing, to assist with daily
activities.

Day Programs:

- Explore adult day programs,
  which offer structured activities
  and socialisation for individuals
  with dementia.

Community Resources:

- Access local and national
  resources, such as the
  Alzheimer's Association, to find
  information, services, and
  support.

Residential Care Options:

- If needed, explore assisted living facilities or memory care units that specialise in dementia care.

Advanced Care Planning:

- Discuss end-of-life wishes and preferences for palliative and hospice care.

Building a supportive network for individuals with dementia involves collaboration and open communication among family members, caregivers, and healthcare professionals. Providing consistent, compassionate care and seeking support from community resources can enhance the quality of life for both the person with dementia and their caregivers.

Communication Strategies

Effective communication with individuals living with dementia is crucial for maintaining their quality of life and ensuring their well-being. Dementia can affect language, comprehension, and expression, making communication challenging. Here are some communication strategies to help improve interactions with dementia patients:

Maintain a Positive and Calm Demeanour:

- Approach the person with a smile and a warm, calm tone to create a positive atmosphere.

- Avoid showing frustration or impatience, as it can agitate the individual.

Establish Eye Contact:

- Make eye contact when speaking to establish a connection and convey your focus on them.

Use Simple and Clear Language:

- Speak in short, simple sentences, using familiar words, and avoiding jargon or complex language.

- Give one instruction at a time to minimise confusion.

Be Patient and Allow Time:

- Give the person time to process and respond to your communication.

- Avoid interrupting or finishing their sentences for them.

Use Nonverbal Communication:

- Use gestures, facial expressions, and body language to help convey your message.

- Use touch, like holding their hand or offering a comforting hug, if appropriate.

Listen Actively:

- Pay close attention to their nonverbal cues, as they may use gestures, expressions, or sounds to communicate.

- Show that you're listening and value their input.

Repeat and Reinforce:

- Repeat key information or questions if necessary to ensure understanding.

- Offer gentle reminders for things like names and places.

Avoid Arguing and Correcting:

- If the person says something inaccurate or holds a false belief, it's usually best to redirect the conversation or validate their feelings rather than correct them.

Ask Simple Questions:

- Ask open-ended questions that require short answers or simple choices rather than complex queries.

Maintain a Structured Routine:

- A consistent daily routine can help with predictability and reduce anxiety. Inform the person about the schedule.

Use Visual Aids:

- Visual aids like pictures, calendars, and signs can help

convey information, schedules, or choices.

Create a Supportive Environment:

- Minimise distractions and noise to create a calm and focused environment for communication.

Encourage Social Interaction:

- Facilitate social interactions and engage the person in conversations with family and friends.

Acknowledge and Validate Emotions:

- Validate their feelings and emotions, even if you don't fully understand the cause.

- Offer empathy and comfort when they are upset or anxious.

Be Flexible:

- Be prepared to adapt your communication approach as the person's needs change with the progression of dementia.

Distract and Redirect:

- If the person becomes upset or anxious, try to distract them with a different topic or activity.

Utilise Memory Aids:

- Create memory aids like memory books or labelled drawers to help with recognition and memory.

Include them in Decision-Making:

- When appropriate, involve them in decision-making regarding their daily activities, clothes, or meals.

Remember that effective communication with dementia patients requires patience and flexibility. Each person is unique, and their communication abilities may change over time. It's essential to adapt your approach to meet their needs and focus on maintaining a respectful and supportive relationship. Additionally, involving caregivers, family members, and healthcare professionals in communication strategies can enhance the overall care and support for individuals with dementia.

Creating a Safe Home Environment

Creating a safe home environment for individuals living with dementia is crucial to prevent accidents, reduce anxiety, and support their overall well-being. Dementia can lead to cognitive and physical challenges, making safety modifications essential. Here are some steps to create a safe home environment:

Remove Hazards:

- Identify and eliminate tripping hazards like loose rugs, clutter, and electrical cords.

- Secure area rugs and use non-slip mats.

- Install safety gates in areas that may be dangerous, such as staircases.

Install Handrails and Grab Bars:

- Install handrails in hallways and on staircases to provide support and reduce the risk of falls.

- Place grab bars in the bathroom near the toilet and shower to assist with balance and mobility.

Proper Lighting:

- Ensure that the home is well-lit, especially in hallways, entryways, and bathrooms.

- Use nightlights to prevent trips and falls in the dark.

Lock Medications and Hazardous Items:

- Secure medications, cleaning products, and other hazardous materials in locked cabinets or drawers.

- Consider installing childproof locks if needed.

Install Door Alarms:

- Install door alarms or chimes on exit doors to alert you when the person tries to leave the house unattended.

Secure Windows:

- Ensure the windows are secure and cannot be easily opened.

- Remove window blinds with looped cords, as they can pose a strangulation risk.

Kitchen Safety:

- Store sharp objects and dangerous kitchen tools out of reach or in locked drawers.

- Use childproof locks on the oven and stove knobs.

- Remove knobs from the stove when not in use.

Label and Colour Code:

- Label drawers and cabinets with pictures or words to help the person locate items.

- Use colour-coded labels for different areas or items to aid in recognition.

Set Up a Memory Care Centre:

- Designate a central area for essential items like keys, phones, glasses, and personal documents to reduce frustration.

Create a Comfortable Bedroom:

- Make the bedroom safe and comfortable, with a comfortable mattress and appropriate bedding.

- Use nightstands with necessary items within easy reach.

Bathroom Modifications:

- Install a raised toilet seat with handles for easier access.

- Use non-slip bath mats and apply non-slip strips in the shower or tub.

- Consider a shower chair for added safety during bathing.

Remove or Lock Firearms:

- If firearms are present in the home, they should be removed or securely locked and stored in a separate location.

Emergency Information:

- Keep a list of emergency contact numbers and medical information easily accessible.

- Place a sign with the person's name and your contact information near the front door.

Wandering Prevention:

- Use door chimes or alarms to alert you when the person attempts to leave.

- If necessary, consider using GPS tracking devices or identification jewellery.

Engage in Activities:

- Provide engaging and stimulating activities to prevent restlessness and wandering.

Regular Safety Assessments:

- Periodically reassess the home environment for potential hazards and make necessary adjustments as the person's condition changes.

Home Security System:

- Consider installing a home security system that includes doorbell cameras and alerts to monitor the person's movements.

Creating a safe home environment for individuals with dementia requires ongoing vigilance and adjustments as their needs change. In addition to physical safety modifications, providing emotional support and maintaining a predictable routine can also contribute to the well-being of individuals living with dementia. It's important to consult with healthcare professionals or occupational therapists for personalised recommendations and to address specific safety concerns related to dementia.

Legal and Financial Planning

Individuals living with dementia require legal and financial planning to guarantee that their preferences are followed, their assets are protected, and their care needs are satisfied. Here are some important steps to take and things to think about:

Legal Planning:

Create Advance Directives:

- Advance directives, including a living will and durable power of attorney for healthcare, allow individuals to specify their medical preferences and designate someone to make healthcare decisions on their behalf.

Establish a Durable Power of Attorney (DPOA):

- A DPOA for finances designates a trusted individual to manage

the person's financial affairs
when they are no longer able to
do so themselves.

Draft a Last Will:

- A will outlines how the
individual's assets should be
distributed after their passing.
It's important to work with an
attorney to ensure that the will is
legally valid.

Set up a Trust:

- A trust can be established to
manage and protect assets,
including property, investments,

and savings, for the benefit of the person with dementia. Trusts can also help avoid probate.

Guardianship and Conservatorship:

- If the person did not designate a DPOA and is deemed unable to make their own decisions, a court may appoint a guardian for their personal and financial affairs.

Review and Update Legal Documents:

- Periodically review and update legal documents to reflect

changing circumstances, preferences, and legal requirements.

Financial Planning:

Assess Financial Resources:

- Take an inventory of the person's financial resources, including income, savings, investments, and insurance policies.

Budgeting:

- Create a comprehensive budget that outlines expenses related to daily living, healthcare, and

other costs associated with
dementia care.

Long-Term Care Planning:

- Explore long-term care options,
  such as in-home care, assisted
  living, or memory care facilities,
  and consider the associated
  costs.

Insurance Coverage:

- Review insurance policies,
  including health, long-term care,
  and life insurance, to
  understand coverage and
  benefits.

Medicaid and VA Benefits:

- Determine eligibility for Medicaid and Veterans Affairs (VA) benefits, as these programmes can help cover the cost of long-term care services.

Protection Against Financial Exploitation:

- Take steps to protect the person from financial exploitation, such as setting up account alerts, monitoring accounts, and educating carers about financial safety.

Consult a Financial Advisor:

- Seek the guidance of a financial advisor or planner who specialises in dementia-related financial planning. They can help with investment strategies, tax planning, and estate planning.

Organise Important Documents:

- Maintain a secure file of important financial documents, including bank statements, tax records, insurance policies, and legal documents.

Monitor and Safeguard Assets:

- Monitor financial accounts for any unusual or unauthorised transactions, and safeguard assets to prevent fraud or scams.

Consider Income Sources:

- Explore options to maximise income sources, such as Social Security benefits and pension plans.

Legal and financial planning for individuals with dementia should ideally begin early, while the person is still capable of making informed decisions. It's crucial to involve an attorney experienced in elder law and a financial advisor who understands the unique challenges associated with dementia. Additionally, open communication among family members is essential to ensure that everyone is aware of the person's wishes and financial situation. Planning can help provide financial security and peace of mind for individuals with dementia and their families.

Chapter 4: Living Well with Dementia

Promoting Quality of Life

The aim of living well with dementia becomes essential for both those who have been diagnosed with the illness and those who provide care for them. It takes a variety of tactics and approaches to encourage independence, uphold mental and physical health, and increase general satisfaction to give dementia patients a great quality of life. The following are essential guidelines for adjusting to dementia:

1. **Early Diagnosis:** Timely diagnosis allows for proper planning and early intervention, enabling individuals and families to make informed decisions about care and support.

2. **Person-Centered Care:** Tailor care and support to the individual's specific needs, preferences, and abilities, respecting their identity and autonomy.

3. **Empowerment:** Encourage individuals with dementia to participate in decisions related to their

care and daily activities, to the extent possible.

4. **Social Engagement:** Maintain social connections with family and friends to combat isolation, depression, and anxiety. Social interactions can provide emotional support and cognitive stimulation.

5. **Physical Activity:** Encourage regular physical activity appropriate to the person's abilities. Physical exercise can help maintain mobility, reduce the risk of falls, and enhance overall well-being.

6. **Mental Stimulation:** Engage in mentally stimulating activities, such as puzzles, memory games, and creative pursuits, to promote cognitive function.

7. **Nutrition and Hydration:** Ensure a balanced diet and adequate hydration. Address any specific dietary needs or restrictions.

8. **Safe Home Environment:** Create a safe home environment by eliminating hazards and providing memory aids, as discussed in a previous response.

9. **Medication Management:**
Carefully manage and monitor medications, and be aware of potential side effects or drug interactions.

10. **Emotional Support:** Provide emotional support to address feelings of anxiety, depression, or frustration. Emotional well-being is vital to living well with dementia.

11. **Routine and Structure:** Establish a structured daily routine to reduce anxiety and provide predictability.

12. **Respite Care:** Arrange for respite care to give caregivers a break from their caregiving responsibilities.

13. **Community Resources:** Access local and national resources, such as dementia support groups and organisations, for information, services, and support.

14. **Cognitive Behavioural Therapy (CBT):** Consider CBT, which can help individuals with dementia cope with emotional challenges and develop strategies for managing symptoms.

15. **Hobbies and Interests:** Encourage participation in hobbies and activities the person enjoys to enhance their sense of purpose and satisfaction.

16. **Sensory Stimulation:** Explore sensory stimulation, such as music therapy or aromatherapy, to promote relaxation and emotional well-being.

17. **Legal and Financial Planning:** Address legal and financial matters to ensure the individual's wishes are respected and assets are protected.

18. **Advance Care Planning:** Discuss end-of-life wishes and

preferences for palliative and hospice care.

The goal of living well with dementia is to preserve an individual's identity, dignity, and quality of life using a variety of strategies. Providing the best care and support throughout the condition entails cooperation between people who have dementia, their carers, and medical professionals.

Engaging in Meaningful Activities

Living successfully with dementia requires taking part in meaningful activities. These pursuits can improve the quality of life, provide dementia patients with a sense of direction, and support their mental and emotional health. The following are some ideas for fulfilling activities for those suffering from dementia:

1. **Reminiscence Therapy:** Encourage individuals to share and reminisce about their life experiences, using photos, mementoes, or family stories

to trigger memories and foster connections.

2. **Art and Creative Expression:** Engage in art activities like painting, drawing, or colouring. Creative expression can be therapeutic and offer an outlet for emotions.

3. **Music Therapy:** Music has a powerful impact on mood and memory. Play favourite songs or musical instruments, or participate in music therapy sessions.

4. **Gardening:** Gardening provides sensory stimulation and a sense of

accomplishment. Planting flowers, herbs, or vegetables in a garden or even potted plants indoors can be fulfilling.

5. **Cooking and Baking:** Simple cooking or baking activities can be enjoyable and engage the senses of taste and smell.

6. **Physical Activity:** Participate in gentle exercises like chair yoga, stretching, or dancing to maintain mobility and physical well-being.

7. **Reading and Storytelling:** Read aloud from books or share stories.

Encourage the individual to read or listen to audiobooks, even if comprehension is limited.

8. **Puzzles and Games:** Engage in puzzles, crossword puzzles, word searches, or board games that challenge the mind and provide a sense of accomplishment.

9. **Sensory Stimulation:** Provide sensory experiences like textured fabrics, scented oils, or tactile materials to stimulate the senses.

10. **Animal Therapy:** Interact with pets or therapy animals, as the

companionship of animals can be comforting and emotionally rewarding.

11. **Nature Walks:** Go for walks in natural surroundings or bring elements of nature indoors, such as birdwatching or indoor plants.

12. **Social Activities:** Organise gatherings with family and friends to encourage social interaction and maintain connections.

13. **Volunteer Work:** Participate in volunteer activities tailored to the person's abilities and interests,

providing a sense of contribution to the community.

14. **Technology and Memory Apps:** Explore technology-based activities, including memory apps and simple tablet games designed for individuals with dementia.

15. **Arts and Crafts:** Engage in arts and crafts, such as knitting, collage, or beadwork, to encourage creativity and self-expression.

16. **Photography:** Use cameras or smartphones to capture everyday

moments, fostering a sense of accomplishment and creativity.

17. **Purposeful Tasks:** Encourage involvement in simple, purposeful tasks like setting the table, folding laundry, or organising items, which provide structure and a sense of achievement.

18. **Multi-Sensory Rooms:** Some care facilities offer multi-sensory rooms with a range of sensory experiences, including lighting effects, soothing sounds, and tactile materials.

19. **Attending Cultural and Community Events:** Visit museums, art galleries, or local community events to promote engagement and exposure to new experiences.

It is paramount to modify exercises according to each person's capabilities and inclinations. When choosing activities, keep dementia's stage in mind, as well as any physical or sensory impairments. Assuring that the activities are pleasurable and meaningful is the main objective since it helps people with dementia feel more purposeful in life and improves their general quality of life.

Nutrition and Exercise

Maintaining a balanced diet and incorporating appropriate exercise into the routine are essential components of living well with dementia. These practices can help improve physical health, cognitive function, and overall well-being. Here are some guidelines for nutrition and exercise for individuals with dementia:

Nutrition:

1. **Balanced Diet:** Encourage a balanced diet that includes a variety of foods from all food groups. Focus on fruits, vegetables, whole grains, lean proteins, and healthy fats.

2. **Hydration:** Ensure that the person with dementia stays well-hydrated. Dehydration can affect cognitive function and overall health.

3. **Regular Meals:** Establish a routine for regular meals and snacks to maintain stable energy levels.

4. **Dietary Supplements:** Consult a healthcare professional to determine if vitamin or mineral supplements are needed.

5. **Food Texture:** Adapt the texture of foods as needed. In later stages of dementia, softer or pureed foods may be necessary to prevent choking.

6. **Finger Foods:** Offer finger foods when dexterity becomes an issue. These can be easier to manage and promote independence.

7. **Favourite Foods:** Include familiar and favourite foods in the diet to make mealtime more enjoyable.

8. **Social Eating:** Encourage social interactions during meals by dining with family and friends whenever possible.

9. **Food Presentation:** Present food attractively, using colourful plates and table settings to stimulate appetite.

10. **Small Portions:** Serve smaller portions to avoid overwhelming the individual and prevent overeating.

11. **Sensory Stimulation:** Use scents and flavours to engage the senses and make meals more enjoyable.

Exercise:

1. **Regular Physical Activity:** Encourage regular physical activity suitable to the individual's capabilities. This can include walking, chair exercises, or stretching.

2. **Balance and Strength Training:** Incorporate exercises to improve balance and strength, which can help prevent falls.

3. **Structured Routine:** Establish a consistent exercise routine to create predictability and structure in the daily schedule.

4. **Safety Precautions:** Ensure a safe exercise environment by removing obstacles and providing necessary support, such as handrails or assistive devices.

5. **Engage in Activities:** Integrate exercise into daily activities, such as gardening or household chores, to make it more enjoyable and purposeful.

6. **Outdoor Activities:** Spend time outdoors when possible to benefit from fresh air and natural surroundings.

7. **Flexibility Exercises:** Include flexibility exercises like gentle yoga or tai chi to improve range of motion.

8. **Social Exercise:** Participate in group exercise classes or involve family members to make exercise a social and enjoyable experience.

9. **Exercise Tracking:** Keep a record of exercise sessions to monitor progress and maintain motivation.

10. **Consult a Professional:** Consult with a physical therapist or healthcare provider to design a personalised exercise programme that suits the individual's needs and abilities.

For those with dementia, maintaining a healthy diet and exercise regimen is crucial to enhancing overall well-being. These activities can promote cognitive function, preserve physical health, and improve the quality of life for dementia patients. Take into consideration the person's physical limitations and the stage of dementia when designing a diet and exercise programme for them.

Medications and Treatments

Managing symptoms and enhancing quality of life with medicine and treatment is a common aspect of living well with dementia. Although the majority of dementias have no known cure, several interventions can help with particular symptoms and problems related to the illness. The following are a few typical drugs and therapies used in dementia care:

Medications:

1. **Cholinesterase Inhibitors:**

   Medications like Donepezil (Aricept), Rivastigmine (Exelon), and Galantamine (Razadyne) are used to improve memory and cognitive function in individuals with Alzheimer's disease.

2. **Memantine (Namenda):**

   Memantine is prescribed to manage moderate to severe Alzheimer's symptoms by regulating glutamate, a neurotransmitter involved in learning and memory.

3. **Antipsychotic Medications:** In some cases, antipsychotic medications may be prescribed to manage severe agitation, aggression, or psychosis, although their use is carefully monitored due to potential side effects.

4. **Antidepressants:** Antidepressants may be used to manage depression and mood disturbances often seen in individuals with dementia.

5. **Anxiolytics:** These medications are prescribed to manage anxiety and

reduce restlessness in individuals with dementia.

Non-Pharmacological Treatments:

1. **Cognitive Stimulation Therapy:** Structured activities, discussions, and exercises designed to stimulate cognitive function and engage individuals with dementia.

2. **Behavioural Interventions:** These approaches focus on managing challenging behaviours by identifying triggers and using strategies to redirect or modify them.

3. **Music Therapy:** Music therapy can help improve mood, reduce anxiety, and provide cognitive stimulation.

4. **Art Therapy:** Engaging in artistic activities can promote self-expression and emotional well-being.

5. **Reminiscence Therapy:** Encouraging individuals to recall and share memories can improve mood and cognition.

6. **Validation Therapy:** Validation therapy emphasises empathy and active listening to connect with the

emotional experiences of individuals with dementia.

7. **Sensory Stimulation:** Using sensory activities, such as aromatherapy or massage, can provide comfort and reduce agitation.

8. **Reality Orientation:** Reality orientation techniques involve consistently providing information about time, place, and people to help individuals with dementia maintain a sense of reality.

9. **Occupational Therapy:** Occupational therapists can help

individuals with dementia maintain independence in daily activities by providing adaptive strategies and assistive devices.

10. **Physical Therapy:** Physical therapy can address mobility and balance issues, reducing the risk of falls.

11. **Speech Therapy:** Speech therapy can help address communication difficulties that may arise as dementia progresses.

12. **Carer Support and Education:** Support and education for caregivers

are crucial in ensuring a high quality of care and improving the overall well-being of the individual with dementia.

It is noteworthy that the selection of drugs and therapies has to be predicated on a comprehensive evaluation conducted by medical experts, considering the kind of dementia, the patient's particular symptoms, and their general state of health. In addition, the course of treatment may change as the illness worsens, and to give the best possible care and assistance, frequent monitoring and modification are required.

Chapter 5: Caregiving Challenges

Role of Caregivers

Caregivers play a vital role in supporting individuals with dementia, but they also face a range of unique challenges. Caring for someone with dementia can be emotionally, physically, and mentally demanding. Among the main difficulties that carers have when providing care are the following:

1. **Emotional Stress:** Carers often experience a wide range of emotions, including sadness, frustration, guilt, and anxiety. Witnessing the decline of

a loved one can be emotionally distressing.

2. **Burnout:** Carers may neglect their well-being, leading to burnout. The demands of caregiving can be relentless, leaving little time for self-care.

3. **Physical Demands:** Providing care, such as assisting with daily activities, lifting, and transferring, can be physically demanding and may lead to carer fatigue and strain.

4. **Financial Burden:** The cost of dementia care, including medications,

medical appointments, home modifications, and long-term care, can place a significant financial burden on caregivers and their families.

5. **Loss of Personal Time:** Caregiving often consumes the caregiver's time, leaving little opportunity for personal pursuits, leisure activities, or work outside the home.

6. **Challenging Behaviours:** Dementia can manifest in challenging behaviours such as aggression, agitation, and wandering, which can be difficult for caregivers to manage.

7. **Social Isolation:** Carers may experience social isolation as they spend more time providing care and less time engaging in social activities.

8. **Communication Difficulties:** Dementia can impair communication, making it challenging for carers to understand and connect with the person they are caring for.

9. **Lack of Information and Support:** Carers may struggle to find reliable information and support, especially if they are unfamiliar with dementia care and available resources.

10. **Grief and Anticipatory Grief:**
Caregivers may experience grief over
the loss of the person they once knew
and anticipatory grief as they
anticipate further decline.

11. **Balancing Responsibilities:** Many
caregivers have multiple
responsibilities, such as work, family,
and their health, which can be difficult
to balance with caregiving.

12. **Sleep Disturbances:** Individuals
with dementia often have sleep
disturbances, which can lead to sleep
deprivation for caregivers.

13. **Role Reversal:** Caregivers may find it emotionally challenging to transition into a role where they are making decisions for the person with dementia who once cared for them.

14. **Safety Concerns:** Caregivers need to continually ensure the safety of the person with dementia, including preventing falls and managing medications.

15. **Lack of Recognition:** Caregivers may feel undervalued and under-recognised for their dedication and hard work.

To address these challenges, caregivers need to seek support and resources. Connecting with dementia support groups, accessing respite care, and consulting healthcare professionals or social workers can provide valuable assistance and relief. Additionally, self-care is essential for caregivers to maintain their well-being, and reaching out to friends and family for help can also ease the burden. Recognising and addressing caregiving challenges is crucial for providing the best possible care to individuals with dementia while taking care of one's own needs.

Managing Caregiver Stress

To guarantee that carers can give dementia patients the greatest care possible while simultaneously preserving their well-being, carer stress must be managed. The following techniques can help carers manage and lower their stress levels:

Seek Support: Connect with support groups, either in-person or online, to share experiences and gain insights from others who are in similar situations.

Respite Care: Arrange for respite care to take breaks from caregiving. This allows caregivers to recharge and reduce burnout.

Set Realistic Expectations: Recognise that caregivers cannot do everything. Set realistic expectations for what can be accomplished each day.

Self-Care: Prioritise self-care by getting adequate sleep, eating well, and engaging in physical activity. Caregivers need to care for themselves to be effective caregivers.

Time Management: Organise tasks and create a schedule to manage caregiving responsibilities efficiently. Time management tools and techniques can help.

Accept Help: Allow friends and family to assist with caregiving tasks. Be specific about what you need, and don't hesitate to accept offers of help.

Educate Yourself: Learn about dementia and caregiving strategies. Understanding the condition can reduce stress and increase confidence in providing care.

Practice Stress Reduction Techniques: Engage in relaxation techniques like deep breathing, meditation, or yoga to manage stress and anxiety.

Stay Connected: Maintain social connections with friends and family. Isolation can exacerbate stress, so nurturing social relationships is important.

Professional Help: Consult with healthcare professionals, therapists, or counsellors to address caregiver stress and emotional well-being.

Take Breaks: Schedule regular breaks and short respites during the day to refresh and reset.

Join a Support Network: Join a caregiver support network to access information, resources, and assistance.

Boundary Setting: Set clear boundaries between caregiving and personal time to prevent caregiver burnout.

Explore Community Resources: Research community resources, such as adult day care services, home health care, or meal delivery programmes, to ease the caregiving load.

Keep a Journal: Documenting thoughts and feelings in a journal can provide an emotional outlet and help caregivers process their experiences.

Practice Patience and Compassion: Understand that dementia can lead to challenging behaviours. Respond to these behaviours with patience, empathy, and a calm demeanour.

Legal and Financial Planning: Address legal and financial matters to ensure the well-being of both the caregiver and the person with dementia.

Express Your Feelings: Share your feelings with a trusted friend or therapist. It's important to express the challenges you face and seek emotional support.

Plan for the Future: Consider long-term care and end-of-life planning, which can help reduce anxiety about future care decisions.

Managing caregiver stress is an ongoing process, and it's crucial to adapt strategies as the caregiving journey evolves. Effective stress management not only benefits caregivers but also enhances the quality of care provided to individuals with dementia. Caregivers should remember that seeking help and support is a sign of strength, not weakness, and is essential for their well-being and the well-being of their loved ones.

Seeking Professional Help

Seeking professional help is an important step for caregivers facing the many challenges of caring for individuals with dementia. Healthcare professionals and therapists can provide guidance, support, and valuable resources to help caregivers navigate the complexities of dementia care. Here are some ways to seek professional help:

1. **Primary Care Physician:** Start by consulting the individual's primary care physician. They can provide an initial assessment, address medical concerns, and offer referrals to specialists when needed.

2. **Specialist Services:** Depending on the type of dementia and specific

challenges, consider consulting specialists such as neurologists, geriatricians, or psychiatrists with expertise in dementia care.

3. **Geriatric Care Manager:** A geriatric care manager can assist in coordinating medical care, providing guidance on long-term care planning, and connecting caregivers with appropriate resources.

4. **Counselling and Therapy:** Individual therapy or counselling can help caregivers manage emotional stress, depression, and anxiety related

to caregiving. Therapists can offer coping strategies and emotional support.

5. **Support Groups:** Many communities have dementia caregiver support groups. Joining these groups provides an opportunity to share experiences, seek advice, and receive emotional support from others in similar situations.

6. **Alzheimer's or Dementia Associations:** Reach out to organisations like the Alzheimer's Association or other dementia-focused

organisations. They often offer information, resources, and support services.

7. **Respite Care Providers:** Respite care services provide temporary relief for caregivers, allowing them to take a break while professionals care for the person with dementia.

8. **Home Health Care Services:** Home health care agencies can provide skilled nursing, therapy, and other medical services in the home, helping carers manage the individual's healthcare needs.

9. **Eldercare Attorneys:** Consult with eldercare attorneys to address legal matters, such as estate planning, guardianship, and advanced care directives.

10. **Financial Advisors:** Financial advisors experienced in eldercare can guide management of the financial aspects of dementia care and long-term care planning.

11. **Social Workers:** Social workers can help with emotional support, connecting caregivers with community

resources, and providing assistance with complex care decisions.

12. **Memory Care Facilities:** If the level of care required becomes too extensive, memory care facilities or assisted living facilities specialising in dementia care can provide professional support.

13. **Hospice and Palliative Care:** In the later stages of dementia, hospice and palliative care services can offer specialised care and support for both the individual with dementia and the caregiver.

14. **Telehealth Services:** In some cases, caregivers can access professional guidance through telehealth services, which offer remote consultations with healthcare providers and therapists.

15. **In-Home Assessments:** Consider arranging an in-home assessment by an occupational therapist or healthcare professional to evaluate the living environment and recommend necessary modifications.

16. **Medication Management:** If medication management becomes complex, consult a pharmacist or

geriatric pharmacist who can offer guidance on drug interactions, side effects, and administration.

17. **Mental Health Services:** For caregivers experiencing severe stress, depression, or anxiety, seeking mental health services from psychologists or psychiatrists is important for their emotional well-being.

It's important for caregivers to proactively seek professional help and not hesitate to reach out for support. Professional guidance can help caregivers better understand dementia, navigate the healthcare system, access community resources, and manage the emotional challenges that come with caregiving. Collaborating with healthcare professionals and specialists is a critical component of providing the best care for individuals with dementia while taking care of the caregiver's well-being.

- Respite Care Options

Respite care provides caregivers with short-term breaks from their caregiving responsibilities, offering much-needed relief and a chance to recharge. Here are various respite care options for caregivers:

1. **In-Home Respite Care:** Trained professionals come to the caregiver's home to provide care for the individual with dementia. They can assist with daily activities, offer companionship, and monitor the person's well-being.

2. **Adult Day Care Centers:** These centres offer structured daytime programmes for individuals with dementia, allowing caregivers to work or take time for themselves while knowing their loved one is in a safe and engaging environment.

3. **Residential Respite Care:** Some memory care facilities or assisted living communities offer short-term stays for individuals with dementia. This option can be beneficial for caregivers who need extended breaks or vacations.

4. **Friends and Family:** Enlist the help of friends and family members who can provide respite care. Loved ones can take turns caring for the individual with dementia, offering caregivers much-needed breaks.

5. **Professional Caregivers:** Hire professional caregivers or certified nursing assistants to provide in-home respite care. Ensure they have experience in dementia care and are well-qualified.

6. **Volunteer Respite Programs:** Some community organisations offer volunteer respite programmes where trained volunteers provide short-term care for individuals with dementia, allowing caregivers time to recharge.

7. **Telehealth Respite Services:** In some cases, caregivers can access

telehealth services to receive professional advice and support, even when taking a break from direct caregiving.

8. **Short-Term Respite Stays:** Some long-term care facilities offer short-term respite stays for individuals with dementia. This can be a valuable option when caregivers need an extended break or have other commitments.

9. **Faith-Based Respite Services:** Religious or faith-based organisations often provide respite care services,

sometimes free of charge, to support caregivers in their communities.

10. **Hospice Respite Care:** For individuals in the later stages of dementia, hospice services may offer respite care to provide relief to caregivers while ensuring the person with dementia receives appropriate end-of-life care.

11. **Vacation Care Programs:** Some vacation care programmes specifically cater to individuals with dementia, allowing caregivers to take a vacation

while their loved one enjoys a safe and engaging environment.

12. **Backup Care Services:** Companies and organisations may offer backup care services, which can provide respite care for employees caring for a family member with dementia.

It is up to carers to look at a range of options and choose the respite care plan that best fits their needs and preferences. Arranging periodic breaks for carers is crucial in preventing burnout, reducing anxiety, and maintaining overall health. Carer contacts should be made with social workers, medical

professionals, and support groups to take
advantage of the community's respite care
resources.

Chapter 6: Dementia and Relationships

Impact on Family Dynamics

Dementia can have a profound effect on family dynamics in several ways, frequently posing difficulties that strain bonds within the family. Dementia frequently affects family dynamics in the following ways:

1. **Role Reversal**: As the person with dementia experiences cognitive decline, roles within the family may shift. Adult children may find themselves taking on more caregiving

responsibilities for their parents, which can lead to feelings of stress, resentment, or guilt. This reversal of roles can disrupt traditional family dynamics and create tension.

2. **Emotional Strain**: Watching a loved one experience cognitive decline can be emotionally challenging for family members. Feelings of sadness, grief, frustration, and helplessness are common. Family members may also experience anticipatory grief as they mourn the loss of the person their loved one once was.

3. **Communication Challenges**:

   Dementia can impair communication skills, making it difficult for the person with dementia to express themselves clearly or understand others. This can lead to frustration and misunderstandings within the family. Family members may need to adjust their communication styles and find alternative ways to connect with their loved ones.

4. **Financial Stress**: Caring for a person with dementia can be expensive, particularly if professional

care services are needed. Financial strain can put additional pressure on family relationships, especially if there are disagreements about how to manage finances or if family members have differing opinions on the best course of action for care.

5. **Social Isolation**: Family caregivers may become socially isolated as they devote more time and energy to caring for their loved one with dementia. This can strain relationships with friends and extended family members who may not understand the

challenges of caregiving or who may not know how to offer support.

6. **Decision-Making**: As the person with dementia becomes less able to make decisions for themselves, family members may need to step in and make decisions on their behalf. This can lead to conflicts among family members if there are disagreements about what is in the best interest of the person with dementia.

7. **Loss of Independence**: Dementia often results in a loss of independence for the person affected, which can be

difficult for both the individual and their family members to accept.

Family dynamics may be impacted as family members grapple with how to balance promoting independence with ensuring the safety and well-being of their loved ones.

All things considered, a family must exercise tolerance, understanding, and open communication when negotiating the problems posed by dementia. Obtaining assistance from medical professionals, support groups, and more resources can aid families in managing the effects of dementia on their interpersonal connections.

Maintaining Connections

Maintaining connections and relationships when a loved one has dementia is crucial for their well-being and the well-being of the family. Here are some strategies to help maintain connections:

1. **Communication Strategies**: Adjust your communication style to accommodate the needs of the person with dementia. Use simple language, speak slowly, and maintain eye

contact. Focus on expressing warmth and empathy, even if the conversation is challenging.

2. **Create Meaningful Activities**: Engage in activities that the person with dementia enjoys and finds meaningful. This could include listening to music, looking at old photographs, or going for a walk together. These activities can help strengthen the bond between family members and provide opportunities for shared experiences.

3. **Reminisce Together**: Sharing experiences from the past helps foster relationships and improve cognitive performance. As the dementia patient shares anecdotes from their history, encourage them to do so while paying attention and joining in on the discussion. Memories can help family members feel more connected and like they belong.

4. **Involve the Person with Dementia in Family Rituals**: Continue to involve the person with dementia in family traditions and

rituals, such as holiday celebrations or family gatherings. Adapt activities to accommodate their abilities and preferences, and focus on creating a sense of inclusion and belonging.

5. **Stay Flexible and Patient**: Understand that dementia can impact he person's ability to engage in social interactions and activities. Be patient and flexible, and adapt your expectations based on the person's current abilities and mood. Focus on creating a supportive and

understanding environment where the person feels comfortable and valued.

6. **Seek Support**: Don't hesitate to reach out for support from healthcare professionals, support groups, or other resources in your community. Caregiving for a loved one with dementia can be challenging, and having a support network can help you navigate the ups and downs of the journey while maintaining connections with your loved one.

7. **Take Care of Yourself**: To preserve your well-being as a carer, never forget

to give self-care priority. Maintaining meaningful connections within the family and providing better assistance for your loved one with dementia will be made possible by taking care of your physical, emotional, and mental health.

Families can continue to foster ties and connections with their loved one who has dementia by putting these strategies into practice and creating a loving and understanding atmosphere. This will improve the loved one's overall health and quality of life.

Coping with Changes in Behaviour

It can be difficult for both the dementia patient and their family members to adjust to behavioural changes brought on by the disease. The following coping mechanisms can be used to handle these relationship changes:

1. **Educate Yourself**: Understanding the behaviours associated with dementia can help family members cope more effectively. Educate yourself about the symptoms and progression of dementia, as well as common behavioural changes that

may occur. This knowledge can help you respond with empathy and patience.

2. **Communicate with Empathy**: When interacting with a person with dementia, approach them with empathy and understanding. Be patient, listen attentively, and respond with kindness. Avoid arguing or correcting the person, as this can escalate the situation and cause distress.

3. **Identify Triggers**: Pay attention to the circumstances or events that

trigger challenging behaviours in the person with dementia. By identifying triggers, you can take steps to minimize them or adjust the environment to reduce stress and agitation.

4. **Establish Routines**: Establishing consistent daily routines can provide structure and predictability for the person with dementia, which can help reduce anxiety and challenging behaviours. Stick to familiar routines for activities such as meals, medication, and bedtime.

5. **Redirect Attention**: When faced with challenging behaviours, gently redirect the person's attention to a different activity or topic. Offer reassurance and distraction to help alleviate their distress.

6. **Practice Self-Care**: Caring for a loved one with dementia can be emotionally and physically demanding. Make sure to prioritize self-care and seek support from other family members, friends, or support groups. Taking breaks and managing

stress will help you cope more effectively with changes in behaviour.

7. **Seek Professional Help**: If challenging behaviours become overwhelming or difficult to manage, don't hesitate to seek help from healthcare professionals. They can offer guidance, support, and interventions to address behavioural symptoms and improve the quality of life for both the person with dementia and their caregivers.

8. **Join Support Groups**: Joining a support group for caregivers of

individuals with dementia can provide valuable emotional support and practical advice. Connecting with others who are going through similar experiences can help you feel less isolated and more empowered to cope with changes in behaviour.

Family members can more effectively negotiate the difficulties of dementia-related behavioural changes while preserving important relationships with their loved ones by using these coping mechanisms and getting help when necessary.

Intimacy and Dementia

It can be difficult to sustain closeness and emotional connection in a relationship when one spouse has dementia, but it is still possible. In the context of dementia, the following advice can help you navigate intimacy:

1. **Communication**: Open and honest communication is key to maintaining intimacy. Even if verbal communication becomes difficult for the person with dementia, non-verbal cues such as touch, eye contact, and facial expressions can still convey love

and affection. Use simple language and expressions of love to reassure your partner.

2. **Physical Touch**: Physical touch can be a powerful way to maintain intimacy and connection. Holding hands, hugging, and cuddling can communicate love and support, even if verbal communication is limited. Be attuned to your partner's preferences and comfort level with physical touch.

3. **Shared Activities**: Engaging in activities together can foster intimacy and create opportunities for

connection. Choose activities that your partner enjoys and can participate in comfortably. This could include listening to music, going for a walk, or simply sitting together and enjoying each other's company.

4. **Adaptation**: As dementia progresses, you may need to adapt your expectations and approaches to intimacy. Focus on finding new ways to connect emotionally and express love and affection. Be patient and flexible as you navigate changes in your relationship.

5. **Seek Support**: Don't hesitate to seek support from healthcare professionals, counsellors, or support groups if you're struggling to navigate intimacy in the context of dementia. These resources can offer guidance, strategies, and emotional support to help you maintain intimacy and connection with your partner.

6. **Respect and Dignity**: Treat your partner with respect and dignity at all times, recognising their autonomy and individuality. Avoid infantilizing or patronising behaviour, and involve

them in decision-making to the extent possible. Respect their boundaries and preferences when it comes to intimacy.

7. **Self-Care**: Remember to prioritise self-care as a caregiver, as caring for a partner with dementia can be emotionally and physically demanding. Take breaks when needed, seek support from friends and family, and engage in activities that bring you joy and relaxation.

Navigating intimacy in the context of dementia requires patience, understanding, and adaptability. By focusing on emotional connection, communication, and shared experiences, you can continue to nurture intimacy and connection with your partner throughout the progression of dementia.

Chapter 7: Dementia in Later Stages

Progression of Symptoms

A person's physical and cognitive abilities deteriorate dramatically as the dementia progresses, and the symptoms intensify. The following are some typical characteristics and symptom progressions seen in the latter stages of dementia:

1. **Severe Memory Impairment**: Memory loss becomes profound, with the individual struggling to recall recent events, recognize familiar faces,

or remember personal information.
Long-term memory may also be
affected, leading to difficulty
remembering significant life events or
personal history.

2. **Communication Challenges**: As
language skills deteriorate,
communication gets harder and
harder. The person could have trouble
speaking, interpreting spoken
language, or keeping up with
conversations. It may become more
crucial to communicate demands and

emotions through nonverbal cues like gestures and facial expressions.

3. **Impaired Judgment and Decision-Making**: Judgment and decision-making abilities deteriorate, leading to poor decision-making and impulsivity. The individual may struggle to understand cause-and-effect relationships or assess risks, which can lead to unsafe behaviours.

4. **Personality and Behavioral Changes**: Changes in personality and behaviour are common in the later

stages of dementia. The individual may become more agitated, irritable, or apathetic. They may also exhibit repetitive behaviours, such as pacing or hand-wringing, or engage in socially inappropriate actions.

5. **Loss of Physical Abilities**: As dementia worsens, physical functioning deteriorates and mobility, coordination, and self-care issues arise. The person could need help with everyday living tasks like eating, dressing, and using the restroom. Additionally, muscle rigidity and

weakness may occur, raising the
possibility of accidents and falls.

6. **Sleep Disturbances**: Sleep
disturbances, such as insomnia or
frequent waking during the night, are
common in the later stages of
dementia. Changes in sleep patterns
can exacerbate cognitive and
behavioural symptoms and contribute
to caregiver stress and fatigue.

7. **Difficulty Swallowing and Eating**:
Swallowing difficulties, known as
dysphagia, may develop in the later
stages of dementia, making it

challenging for the individual to eat and drink safely. This can lead to weight loss, dehydration, and an increased risk of aspiration pneumonia.

8. **Loss of Awareness and Recognition**: The individual may become less aware of their surroundings and less responsive to stimuli. They may have difficulty recognizing familiar people, places, or objects, leading to feelings of disorientation and confusion.

9. **Increased Dependence on Caregivers**: As the symptoms of dementia worsen, the individual becomes increasingly dependent on caregivers for support and assistance. Caregivers may need to provide around-the-clock care to ensure the safety and well-being of the person with dementia.

In general, a substantial reduction in cognitive and physical functioning is a hallmark of the later stages of dementia, which results in severe alterations to the person's abilities and behaviour. During this difficult stage of the disease, sustaining the person with dementia's dignity and quality of life requires providing them with caring care and support.

Palliative and Hospice Care

Hospice and palliative care play a crucial role in an individual's overall care plan during the later stages of dementia, when their quality of life has been considerably compromised and their condition has significantly deteriorated. How these methods can be useful is as follows:

1. **Palliative Care**: The primary objective of palliative care is to enhance the quality of life for the dementia patient and their family by relieving the symptoms and stress associated with a serious illness. Palliative care in the setting of dementia may entail attending to emotional, social, and spiritual needs in addition to symptom management for pain, agitation, and discomfort. In addition to other treatments targeted at treating the condition, palliative care can be incorporated into the

overall care plan at any stage of dementia.

2. **Hospice Care**: Hospice care is a specialised form of palliative care designed for individuals with a terminal illness who are nearing the end of life. In the context of dementia, hospice care may be appropriate in the later stages of the disease when the individual's condition has advanced significantly and life expectancy is limited. Hospice care focuses on providing comfort and dignity to the person with dementia in their final

days or weeks, with an emphasis on pain management, symptom control, and emotional support. Hospice services can be provided in various settings, including the individual's home, a hospice facility, or a nursing home.

3. **Comfort and Support**: Both palliative and hospice care prioritise the individual's comfort and well-being, aiming to alleviate suffering and promote dignity in the face of a progressive and incurable disease. Caregivers trained in

palliative and hospice care techniques can provide specialised support tailored to the unique needs of individuals with dementia and their families, offering compassionate care and guidance throughout the end-of-life journey.

4. **Emotional and Spiritual Care**: Palliative and hospice care teams include professionals such as nurses, social workers, chaplains, and counsellors who are trained to address the emotional and spiritual needs of individuals with dementia and their

families. These professionals provide counselling, support groups, and spiritual guidance to help individuals and families cope with the challenges of dementia and find meaning and comfort in the final stages of life.

5. **Family Support**: Palliative and hospice care also offer support and resources for family members and caregivers,recognising the significant emotional, physical, and practical burdens they may face. Caregivers are encouraged to participate in care planning, express their concerns and

preferences, and access respite care and support services to help alleviate caregiver stress and burnout.

All things considered, palliative and hospice care are crucial in helping people with dementia and their families in the latter stages of the illness by offering comfort, dignity, and support. These methods aid in ensuring that people with dementia receive compassionate, respectful, and dignified end-of-life care that respects their values and way of life by emphasising quality of life and holistic care.

End-of-Life Decisions

Making decisions about a loved one's end of life can be emotionally taxing, but it's crucial to make sure that their desires are honoured and that they receive compassionate care that aligns with their moral principles. When making decisions about someone's death in the later stages of dementia, keep the following in mind:

1. **Advance Care Planning**:
   Encourage your loved one to engage in advance care planning while they are still able to communicate their preferences and wishes. This may

involve discussing their values, goals of care, and preferences for medical treatments, including resuscitation, hospitalisation, and life-sustaining interventions. Documenting these preferences in advance directives or living wills can guide medical decision-making in the later stages of dementia.

2. **Quality of Life**: Focus on maintaining your loved one's quality of life and ensuring that their care aligns with their values and goals. Consider factors such as comfort,

dignity, and autonomy when making
decisions about medical treatments,
interventions, and end-of-life care.
Palliative and hospice care can help
manage symptoms and provide
comfort and support in the final stages
of dementia.

3. **Respecting Autonomy**: Respect
your loved one's autonomy and right
to make decisions about their care to
the extent possible, even as their
cognitive abilities decline. Involve
them in decision-making to the extent
that they are able, and honour their

preferences and choices whenever feasible. Consider their past expressions of values and wishes when making decisions on their behalf.

4. **Family Discussions**: Have open and honest discussions with family members about end-of-life decisions for your loved one with dementia. Share information, concerns, and preferences openly, and work together to make decisions that prioritise your loved one's well-being and dignity. Consider seeking guidance from healthcare professionals, social

workers, or spiritual advisors to facilitate family discussions and decision-making.

5. **Medical Proxy or Power of Attorney**: If your loved one is unable to make decisions for themselves due to advanced dementia, designate a trusted individual as their medical proxy or power of attorney for healthcare. This person will be responsible for making medical decisions on behalf of your loved one based on their known preferences and best interests.

6. **Regular Reevaluation**:

   Continuously reevaluate your loved one's medical condition, treatment options, and goals of care as their dementia progresses. Be prepared to adjust care plans and treatment decisions based on changes in their condition and evolving needs and preferences.

7. **Emotional Support**: Seek emotional support for yourself and your family members as you navigate end-of-life decisions for your loved one with dementia. Counselling,

support groups, and spiritual guidance can provide comfort, guidance, and reassurance during this challenging time.

Making end-of-life decisions for a loved one with dementia requires sensitivity, compassion, and collaboration among family members and healthcare providers. By prioritising your loved one's values, wishes, and quality of life, you can ensure that they receive dignified and compassionate care in the final stages of dementia.

Grief and Loss

Being a carer for someone who has dementia, especially in the latter stages when their condition has drastically deteriorated, is bound to involve experiencing grief and loss. Family members and carers may experience grief and loss in the following ways:

1. **Anticipatory Grief**: Family members often experience anticipatory grief as they witness the gradual decline of their loved one with dementia. Anticipatory grief involves mourning the loss of the person as

they once were, as well as anticipating the loss of their future abilities and memories. This can be a prolonged and complex grieving process that occurs before the person's death.

2. **Ambiguous Loss**: Dementia can result in ambiguous loss, where the person is physically present but mentally or emotionally unavailable. Family members may grieve the loss of their loved one's former personality, memories, and abilities, even while they are still alive. Ambiguous loss can be challenging to navigate, as there is

no clear endpoint to the grieving process.

3. **Role Reversal**: Caring for a loved one with dementia often involves significant role reversal, with adult children becoming caregivers for their parents. This reversal of roles can lead to feelings of grief and loss as family members mourn the changing dynamics of their relationship and the loss of their loved one's independence and autonomy.

4. **Multiple Losses**: As dementia progresses, family members may

experience multiple losses, including the loss of communication, companionship, and shared memories. Each stage of the disease may bring new losses and challenges to cope with, leading to cumulative grief over time.

5. **Disenfranchised Grief**: Grief related to dementia may be disenfranchised, meaning it is not openly acknowledged or validated by society. Family members may feel isolated or misunderstood in their grief, particularly if others fail to

recognise the impact of dementia on their lives and relationships.

6. **Complicated Grief**: Some family members may experience complicated grief, which is characterised by intense and prolonged feelings of sadness, guilt, or anger that interfere with daily functioning. Complicated grief may occur when there are unresolved issues or conflicts in the relationship with the person who has dementia, or when the caregiver has difficulty accepting the inevitability of their loved one's decline.

7. **Self-Care and Support**: Family members and caregivers need to prioritise self-care and seek support to cope with the grief and loss associated with dementia. This may involve talking to a counsellor or therapist, joining a support group for caregivers, or engaging in self-care activities that promote emotional well-being.

In addition to finding support and comfort in their shared experiences, family members and carers can better negotiate the emotional challenges of caring for a loved one with dementia by identifying and expressing their feelings of sadness and loss.

Chapter 8: Dementia-Friendly Communities

Creating Inclusive Environments

Communities that are dementia-friendly are those that are inclusive, encouraging, and easily accessible to those who are caring for those who have dementia and to them. The following are some essential tactics for developing dementia-friendly communities:

1. **Education and Awareness**: Raise awareness and promote understanding of dementia within the community. Educate community

members, businesses, organizations, and service providers about the challenges faced by individuals living with dementia and their caregivers. Offer training programs and workshops to help people recognize the signs of dementia and learn how to interact with and support individuals affected by the disease.

2. **Accessible Environment**: Design public spaces and facilities to be accessible and easy to navigate for individuals with dementia. This may include clear signage, contrasting

colours, uncluttered pathways, and ergonomic design features. Ensure that public transportation, parks, shops, and other community resources are accessible to individuals with mobility issues or cognitive impairments.

3. **Social Inclusion**: Promote social inclusion and community engagement for individuals living with dementia. Create opportunities for social interaction, participation, and meaningful engagement in community life. This may involve organizing social

activities, support groups, recreational programs, and cultural events specifically tailored to the needs and interests of individuals with dementia.

4. **Supportive Services**: Offer a range of supportive services and resources to help individuals with dementia and their caregivers navigate daily life. This may include home care services, respite care, memory cafes, adult day programs, and caregiver support groups. Ensure that these services are easily accessible, affordable, and

responsive to the needs of the community.

5. **Dementia-Friendly Businesses**: Encourage local businesses to become dementia-friendly by training staff to recognize and respond to the needs of customers with dementia. Guide how businesses can create a welcoming and supportive environment, such as offering assistance with shopping, providing quiet spaces, and accommodating special needs.

6. **Community Partnerships**: Foster collaboration and partnerships

between local government, businesses, healthcare providers, nonprofit organizations, and community groups to create dementia-friendly initiatives and programs. Pool resources, share best practices, and coordinate efforts to improve the overall quality of life for individuals with dementia and their caregivers.

7. **Advocacy and Policy**: Advocate for policies and legislation that support the rights and needs of individuals living with dementia and their caregivers. This may include

advocating for dementia-friendly design standards, funding for supportive services, and policies to protect the rights and dignity of people with dementia.

Communities may build conditions that allow people with dementia to remain involved, independent, and connected to their community for as long as feasible by applying these techniques and cultivating an inclusive and supportive culture.

Community Support Services

By offering information, help, and support to people with dementia and their carers, community support services are essential to the development of dementia-friendly communities. The following are some essential community services that help create dementia-friendly communities:

1. **Memory Cafés**: Memory cafés are social gatherings designed specifically for individuals living with dementia and their carers. These cafés offer a relaxed and supportive environment where participants can socialise, share

experiences, and participate in engaging activities. Memory cafés promote social inclusion and reduce feelings of isolation among individuals affected by dementia.

2. **Caregiver Support Groups**: Caregiver support groups provide a forum for caregivers to connect with others who are experiencing similar challenges and share practical advice, emotional support, and coping strategies. These groups offer a safe space for caregivers to express their feelings, ask questions, and access

information and resources relevant to
caregiving.

3. **Respite Care Services**: Respite care
services offer temporary relief to
caregivers by providing professional
care and supervision for individuals
with dementia. This allows caregivers
to take breaks, attend to their own
needs, and recharge, knowing that
their loved one is in safe hands.
Respite care services may be offered
in-home, at adult day centres, or
through residential respite programs.

4. **Home Care Services**: Home care services assist with activities of daily living, such as bathing, dressing, meal preparation, and medication management, for individuals living with dementia who wish to remain in their own homes. Home care services can help promote independence, dignity, and quality of life for individuals with dementia while providing much-needed support to family carers.

5. **Transportation Services**: Transportation services ensure that

individuals with dementia can access essential services, community resources, and social activities safely and reliably. Accessible transportation options, such as door-to-door transportation or volunteer driver programmes, help individuals with dementia maintain their mobility and independence.

6. **Educational Programmes and Workshops**: Educational programmes and workshops provide information, guidance, and practical skills training to individuals living

with dementia, caregivers, and community members. These programmes cover topics such as dementia awareness, communication strategies, behaviour management, and self-care, empowering participants to better understand and navigate the challenges of dementia.

7. **Information and Referral Services**: Information and referral services connect individuals affected by dementia and their caregivers with relevant resources, services, and support networks in the community.

These services provide guidance, advocacy, and assistance in accessing healthcare, financial assistance, legal resources, and other essential support. Communities may foster a friendly and inclusive atmosphere that improves the well-being and quality of life of people with dementia and their carers by providing a wide range of community support services. These programmes guarantee that people with dementia can continue to be engaged and active members of their communities while also fostering independence, dignity, and social involvement.

Promoting Awareness and Education

To create inclusive, understanding communities that are sensitive to the needs of both carers and those living with dementia, dementia awareness and education must be promoted. The following are some tactics for raising community awareness and educating people about dementia:

1. **Public Awareness Campaigns**: Launch public awareness campaigns to raise awareness about dementia, its symptoms, and its impact on individuals and families. Utilize

various channels such as print media, social media, radio, television, and community events to disseminate information and reach a wide audience.

2. **Community Workshops and Training**: Offer community workshops, seminars, and training sessions to educate community members, businesses, organizations, and service providers about dementia. Topics may include recognizing the signs of dementia, effective communication strategies,

dementia-friendly design principles, and understanding the experiences of individuals living with dementia and their caregivers.

3. **Dementia Friends Programs**: Implement Dementia Friends programs, which are initiatives aimed at raising awareness and changing perceptions about dementia at the grassroots level. Dementia Friends programs provide information and training to community members, encouraging them to become dementia-friendly allies who support

and advocate for individuals living with dementia in their communities.

4. **School Education Programs**: Introduce dementia education programs in schools and educational institutions to teach students about dementia, reduce stigma, and promote empathy and understanding towards individuals affected by the disease. These programs can help foster a culture of compassion and inclusion among future generations.

5. **Healthcare Provider Training**: Provide training and professional

development opportunities for healthcare providers, including physicians, nurses, social workers, and allied health professionals, to enhance their knowledge and skills in dementia care. This includes training on early detection, diagnosis, treatment, and management of dementia, as well as communication techniques and person-centred care approaches.

6. **Community Partnerships and Collaborations**: Foster partnerships and collaborations between local government, healthcare providers,

nonprofit organizations, businesses, schools, and community groups to collectively promote awareness and education about dementia. Pool resources, share expertise, and coordinate efforts to reach diverse segments of the community and maximize impact.

7. **Cultural Competence and Diversity**: Ensure that awareness and education initiatives are culturally sensitive, inclusive, and accessible to individuals from diverse backgrounds, including different ethnicities,

languages, and socio-economic groups. Tailor educational materials and programs to reflect the cultural and linguistic diversity of the community and address unique cultural beliefs and attitudes towards dementia.

8. **Continued Engagement and Evaluation**: Maintain ongoing engagement with the community and regularly evaluate the effectiveness of awareness and education initiatives. Solicit feedback from community members, monitor participation rates,

and assess changes in knowledge, attitudes, and behaviours related to dementia over time. Use this information to refine and improve future efforts.

Communities may be made more inclusive and dementia-friendly for everyone if we prioritise raising awareness and providing education about dementia. By doing this, we can help people living with dementia and their carers feel more understood, empathetic, and supported.

Chapter 9: Research and Advances

Current Research Efforts

The current focus of dementia research is on many topics with the ultimate goal of understanding dementia's underlying causes, creating efficient treatments, enhancing care, and eventually discovering a cure. Here are some important fields of study and current developments:

1. **Biological Mechanisms**:

    Researchers are investigating the biological mechanisms involved in the development and progression of dementia, including the role of genetics, brain changes, inflammation, and protein abnormalities. Advances in neuroimaging techniques, such as positron emission tomography (PET) and functional magnetic resonance imaging (fMRI), allow researchers to study brain structure and function in greater detail.

2. **Genetic Factors**: Genetic studies are identifying genetic risk factors and susceptibility genes associated with dementia, particularly Alzheimer's

disease. Genome-wide association studies (GWAS) and next-generation sequencing technologies have led to the discovery of novel genetic variants implicated in dementia, providing insights into disease mechanisms and potential therapeutic targets.

3. **Biomarker Discovery**: Biomarkers are biological indicators that can be measured in the body and used to diagnose, monitor, and predict the progression of dementia. Researchers are identifying and validating biomarkers for dementia, including

cerebrospinal fluid biomarkers,

blood-based markers, and imaging

biomarkers, to improve early

detection and diagnosis.

4. **Drug Development**:

Pharmaceutical companies and

academic researchers are developing

new drugs and therapeutic approaches

for treating dementia. Targeted

therapies aimed at reducing amyloid

plaques, tau tangles,

neuroinflammation, and other

pathological processes associated with

dementia are under investigation in

clinical trials. Other approaches focus on enhancing cognitive function, neuroprotection, and symptom management.

5. **Non-Pharmacological Interventions**: Non-pharmacological interventions, such as cognitive training, physical exercise, social engagement, and lifestyle modifications, are being studied for their potential to prevent or delay the onset of dementia, as well as improve cognitive function and quality of life in individuals with

dementia. These interventions may
have neuroprotective effects and
promote brain health through various
mechanisms.

6. **Precision Medicine**: Precision
   medicine approaches aim to tailor
   treatment strategies to the individual
   characteristics of each patient,
   including genetic, biological, and
   clinical factors. Researchers are
   exploring personalized medicine
   approaches for dementia, including
   the use of biomarkers to stratify
   patients into subgroups based on

disease subtype, severity, and treatment response.

7. **Caregiver Support and Interventions**: Research is also focusing on developing interventions to support caregivers of individuals with dementia. These interventions may include caregiver education programs, respite care services, support groups, and technological solutions to assist with caregiving tasks and alleviate caregiver burden.

8. **Healthcare Delivery and Policy**: Research efforts are examining

healthcare delivery models, policy initiatives, and public health strategies to improve dementia care, increase access to services, and reduce disparities in diagnosis and treatment. These efforts aim to promote earlier detection, facilitate timely intervention, and enhance the overall quality of care for individuals with dementia and their families.

In general, current dementia research initiatives are expanding our knowledge of the illness, finding new therapeutic targets, and enhancing support and care for those with dementia and those who care for them. The advancement of dementia prevention, treatment, and eventually a cure depends heavily on collaborative research projects including multidisciplinary teams of scientists, physicians, carers, and people with lived experience of dementia.

Potential Breakthroughs

The goal of current dementia research is to build more effective treatments, better care and support for people with dementia and their carers, and an understanding of the underlying causes of the disease. These goals are centred around many major areas. Here are a few possible discoveries and study areas:

1. **Early Detection and Diagnosis**: Researchers are exploring biomarkers and imaging techniques that may help identify individuals at risk of developing dementia at an earlier stage. Early detection allows for timely intervention and treatment, potentially slowing the progression of the disease.

2. **Precision Medicine**: Advances in genetics and genomics are leading to

personalised approaches to dementia
care. Researchers are studying genetic
risk factors and gene-environment
interactions to develop targeted
therapies tailored to individual
patient's unique genetic profiles.

3. **Drug Development**: There is
ongoing research into new drug
targets and therapeutic approaches for
dementia, including Alzheimer's
disease and other forms of dementia.
Clinical trials are testing novel drugs
that target amyloid plaques, tau
tangles, neuroinflammation, and other

pathological mechanisms associated with dementia.

4. **Non-Pharmacological Interventions**:

   Non-pharmacological interventions such as cognitive training, physical exercise, social engagement, and lifestyle modifications are being investigated for their potential to improve cognitive function, delay cognitive decline, and enhance quality of life for individuals with dementia.

5. **Technology and Innovation**:

   Technology-based interventions such

as digital therapeutics, virtual reality, wearable devices, and smartphone apps are being developed to support dementia care, monitor disease progression, and enhance cognitive function and daily functioning for individuals with dementia.

6. **Caregiver Support and Interventions**: Research is focusing on developing interventions and support programmes to address the needs of family carers of individuals with dementia. These programmes aim to reduce caregiver burden, stress,

and depression, and improve carer coping skills, resilience, and quality of life.

7. **Brain Health and Prevention**: There is growing interest in promoting brain health and implementing preventive strategies to reduce the risk of dementia. Research is examining lifestyle factors such as diet, exercise, sleep, cognitive stimulation, and social engagement, as well as vascular risk factors, to identify modifiable factors that may help prevent or delay the onset of dementia.

8. **Global Collaboration and Knowledge Sharing**: International collaborations and initiatives are fostering cooperation among researchers, clinicians, policymakers, and stakeholders to accelerate progress in dementia research and innovation. These collaborations aim to share data, resources, best practices, and research findings to advance our understanding and treatment of dementia on a global scale.

Even if discoveries in the field of dementia research are still being made, continuous efforts are opening the door to fresh perspectives, therapies, and methods of providing dementia care that could ultimately lead to better results and a higher standard of living for those who are affected by the disease as well as their loved ones.

Hope for the Future

Prospects for dementia research and advancements are very promising. Here are a few causes for hope:

1. **Advancements in Early Detection**: Researchers are making progress in identifying biomarkers and other indicators that may allow for earlier detection of dementia, even before symptoms appear. Early detection could lead to interventions that slow or halt the progression of the disease.

2. **Precision Medicine Approaches**: Personalised medicine approaches are being explored, tailoring treatments to individuals based on their genetic makeup, lifestyle factors, and other

personalised characteristics. This
could lead to more effective
treatments with fewer side effects.

3. **Diverse Therapeutic Targets**:
   There's a growing understanding of
   the complex underlying mechanisms
   of dementia, leading to the
   identification of multiple therapeutic
   targets. Researchers are exploring a
   range of approaches, including
   targeting amyloid plaques, tau tangles,
   neuroinflammation, and synaptic
   dysfunction.

4. **Lifestyle Interventions**: Studies have shown that certain lifestyle interventions, such as regular physical exercise, healthy diet, cognitive stimulation, social engagement, and adequate sleep, may help reduce the risk of dementia and slow cognitive decline. These interventions offer accessible and cost-effective strategies for dementia prevention and management.

5. **Technological Innovations**: Advances in technology, including artificial intelligence, wearable

devices, digital therapeutics, and
telemedicine, are revolutionising
dementia care and support. These
technologies have the potential to
enhance early detection, monitoring,
intervention, and support for
individuals with dementia and their
caregivers.

6. **Global Collaboration and
   Funding**: There's growing
   recognition of the global impact of
   dementia and the need for
   collaboration among researchers,
   clinicians, policymakers, and

stakeholders worldwide. International initiatives and funding efforts are fueling research and innovation in dementia prevention, treatment, and care on a global scale.

7. **Empowering Caregivers**: There's increasing recognition of the vital role that family caregivers play in supporting individuals with dementia. Efforts to support and empower caregivers through education, training, respite care, and community resources are helping improve caregiver well-being and quality of life.

8. **Changing Attitudes and Awareness**: There's a growing movement to raise awareness, reduce stigma, and promote understanding of dementia in society. Initiatives such as Dementia Friends programmes, public education campaigns, and community outreach efforts are helping change attitudes and perceptions about dementia, fostering a more dementia-friendly and supportive society.

Even if there is always more to be done, these developments and initiatives give optimism for the future of dementia assistance and care. There's hope that with sustained research, creativity, cooperation, and advocacy, we can improve the quality of life and outcomes for people with dementia and their families significantly.

Glossary

Key Terms and Definitions

Dementia is a complex condition with numerous key terms and definitions. Here are some essential terms and their definitions associated with dementia:

1. **Dementia:** Dementia is an overarching term used to describe a range of cognitive impairments that interfere with a person's daily functioning and quality of life. It is not a specific disease but a syndrome

caused by various underlying conditions.

2. **Alzheimer's Disease:** Alzheimer's disease is the most common cause of dementia. It is a progressive brain disorder characterised by the accumulation of amyloid plaques and tau tangles, leading to memory loss and cognitive decline.

3. **Vascular Dementia:** Vascular dementia is caused by impaired blood flow to the brain, often due to stroke or small blood vessel damage, resulting in cognitive deficits.

4. **Lewy Body Dementia:** Lewy body dementia is characterised by the presence of abnormal protein deposits (Lewy bodies) in the brain, leading to cognitive decline, visual hallucinations, and motor symptoms similar to Parkinson's disease.

5. **Frontotemporal Dementia:** Frontotemporal dementia is a group of disorders that primarily affect the frontal and temporal lobes of the brain, leading to changes in behaviour, personality, and language abilities.

6. **Mild Cognitive Impairment (MCI):** MCI is a condition characterised by cognitive decline that is more noticeable than expected for an individual's age but is not severe enough to be classified as dementia.

7. **Cognitive Impairment:** Cognitive impairment refers to difficulties in thinking, memory, problem-solving, and other cognitive functions that can range from mild to severe.

8. **Neurodegenerative Disease:** Neurodegenerative diseases are conditions in which nerve cells

(neurons) in the brain and spinal cord gradually die, leading to a decline in cognitive and physical function. Alzheimer's, Parkinson's, and Huntington's diseases are examples.

9. **Mini-Mental State Examination (MMSE):** The MMSE is a brief 30-point questionnaire used to assess cognitive impairment and screen for dementia. It evaluates various cognitive functions, including memory, attention, and language.

10. **Caregiver:** A caregiver is an individual who provides physical,

emotional, and practical support to someone with dementia, assisting with daily activities and ensuring their well-being.

11. **Activities of Daily Living (ADLs):** ADLs are fundamental self-care tasks necessary for independent living, such as bathing, dressing, eating, and mobility.

12. **Instrumental Activities of Daily Living (IADLs):** IADLs are more complex daily tasks that are essential for functioning in society, including

managing finances, cooking, and using transportation.

13. **Sundowning:** Sundowning is a phenomenon in which individuals with dementia experience increased confusion, agitation, and behavioural changes, often worsening in the late afternoon and evening.

14. **Delirium:** Delirium is a sudden and severe state of confusion and disorientation that can occur in individuals with dementia, often due to infections, medication side effects,

or other underlying medical conditions.

15. **Respite Care:** Respite care provides temporary relief to the primary caregivers of individuals with dementia, allowing them to take a break from caregiving responsibilities.

These are some of the key terms associated with dementia, but the field of dementia care and research is extensive, and there are many more specialised terms and concepts used in the assessment, diagnosis, and management of the condition.